Glossary of
Histopathological Terms

Under the General Editorship of

F. J. BAKER, F.I.M.L.T., F.I.S.T.

Fellow of the Royal Microscopical Society;
Senior Chief Technician, Department of Pathology,
Brompton Hospital, London:
Associate Lecturer in Bacteriology,
Paddington Technical College, London

Glossary of
Histopathological
Terms

JOHN W. LAW, F.I.M.L.T.

*Senior Chief Technician, Department
of Pathology, Chelsea Hospital for
Women, London*

H. JOHN OLIVER, A.I.M.L.T.

*Senior Chief Technician, Department
of Morbid Anatomy, The London Hospital*

London
Butterworths

ENGLAND: BUTTERWORTH & CO. (PUBLISHERS) LTD.
                LONDON: 88 Kingsway, WC2B 6AB

AUSTRALIA: BUTTERWORTHS PTY. LTD.
                SYDNEY: 586 Pacific Highway, 2067
                MELBOURNE: 343 Little Collins Street, 3000
                BRISBANE: 240 Queen Street, 4000

CANADA: BUTTERWORTH & CO. (CANADA) LTD.
                TORONTO: 14 Curity Avenue, 374

NEW ZEALAND: BUTTERWORTHS OF NEW ZEALAND LTD.
                WELLINGTON: 26–28 Waring Taylor Street, 1

SOUTH AFRICA: BUTTERWORTH & CO. (SOUTH AFRICA) (PTY) LTD.
                DURBAN: 152–154 Gale Street

Suggested U.D.C. Number: 616–091·8 (038)

ISBN 0 407 72730 2

Printed in Great Britain by Redwood Press Limited
Trowbridge, Wiltshire

Preface

The primary object of this book is to present, in alphabetical form, a glossary of terms likely to be encountered by workers in the field of histopathology. It is designed to appeal to a broad spectrum of those interested in the subject, from the veriest beginner to the fully competent histologist. No claim is made that the work is comprehensive: inevitably omissions occur, perhaps unpardonable in the view of some specialists; and conversely, the inclusion of certain items may to others appear indefensible. We feel that such a work is bound to reflect our own individual foibles and preferences, and have endeavoured to present, in everyday laboratory language and without undue esoteric emphases, a source of reference that may provide the basic information and at the same time stimulate the reader to further study.

We acknowledge our indebtedness to numerous friends and colleagues for their assistance, and especially to Mr. Kenneth V. Swettenham of The London Hospital for his help in the realms of histochemistry and microscopy and, in view of the book's lengthy gestation, to our respective long-suffering wives.

J. W. L.
H. J. O.

A

Aberration, chromatic

An optical defect of a lens, whereby unequal refraction of white light causes its emergent constituent rays to form different points of focus for each component colour, the blue—violet rays of shorter wavelength being refracted to a greater degree than the red—orange ones. The fault may be corrected in microscopy, at least in part, by incorporation into the optical system of a negative lens which, in combination with the positive lens, constitutes an achromatic objective. This will give correction for two colours, usually red and blue. Further correction may be achieved by incorporating fluorspar into the lens system, which virtually eliminates chromatic aberration. Such a lens is described as apochromatic.

Aberration, spherical

An intrinsic property of a convex lens whereby there is excessive refraction from the periphery, giving rise to multiple foci and resultant blurred images. The fault may be corrected by the use of a compound lens system.

Abrasive powder (levigated alumina, white bauxilite, etc.)

Used as a lapping compound for honing microtome knives on plate glass. Obtainable in various grades of coarseness, these powders are made into a paste with water or paraffin oil. The use of abrasive powders allows all stages of honing to be carried out on one hone merely by changing the grade of powder as required.

Accelerator

A substance used to enhance metallic impregnation of tissues. These compounds are essentially accentuators (q.v.), but the name is confined to hypnotics such as chloral hydrate and veronal.

1

Accentuator

A substance which enhances the selectivity or intensity of a stain, which already possesses a limited affinity for certain tissue elements. Common examples are borax in toluidine blue and methylene blue solutions, and phenol in solutions of basic fuchsin and auramine.

See also Accelerator, Mordants.

Acetal phosphatides

Compound lipids structurally resembling phospholipids, but instead of two of the hydroxyl groups of glycerol being each bound to a fatty acid, they are together bound to a single fatty aldehyde by acetal linkage. The third hydroxyl group, as in all the phospholipids, is bound to the phosphoric acid–nitrogen complex.

Their demonstration is based on the liberation of aldehydes by short hydrolysis with mercuric chloride and subsequent colouration with Schiff's reagent.

Acetic acid ($CH_3.COOH$)

A colourless corrosive liquid with a pungent smell; it is a fatty acid, mp $16.6°C$, bp $118.1°C$; solidifies at low temperatures to 'glacial acetic acid'.

Its uses in histology include (1) fixation: it precipitates nucleoproteins but not cytoplasmic proteins. Rarely used alone, it figures as a constituent of such well-known fixatives as Carnoy, Bouin, Zenker, and Susa; (2) staining: it is incorporated as an accentuator in dye solutions, notably haematoxylin, in order to promote more specific staining, and is used as a differentiating fluid in several techniques, for instance, Leishman and Nile blue for neutral fats.

Acetone ($CH_3.CO.CH_3$)

A highly inflammable fluid, whose uses in histology include (1) fixation, for instance, in the study of enzymes; (2) dehydration, of both tissues and sections as an alternative to alcohol; (3) stain solution, especially the lipid stains; and (4) differentiation, for example, Gram techniques.

Acetylation

A blocking technique whereby substances possessing 1:2 glycol groups (carbohydrates) are rendered non-reactive to the periodic acid-Schiff reaction. Acetic acid or acetic anhydride has been employed for this purpose. Acetylation may be reversed by treatment with dilute alkali and the PAS reaction restored.

See also Blocking.

Achromatic lens

This in fact consists of a pair of lenses, one of flint, the other of crown glass, and is devised to eliminate chromatic aberration (q.v.).

2

Achromatic spindle

Fine filaments which appear to radiate from the centrioles during the first stage of mitosis (q.v.) and upon which the chromosomes arrange themselves during metaphase.

Acid dye

A stain compound whose colouring property is to be found in its acid component, which property is derived from the acid chromophoric and auxochromic groups therein contained. Such dyes are in fact salts of a colour acid, often the sodium salt, sometimes the calcium, potassium, or ammonium salt, and have usually, but not invariably, an affinity for the more basic tissue components.

Examples of acid dyes in common use are: eosin, orange G, acid fuchsin, light green.

See also Basic dye.

Acid formaldehyde haematin (formalin pigment)

A dark-brown or black, doubly-refractile, granular or amorphous pigment occurring in blood-containing tissues when these are fixed in formalin at an acid pH. In sections it is distributed throughout, is extracellular, and is most profuse inside and around blood vessels. It is insoluble in strong acids, but may be extracted by alkaline-alcohol. or better, by saturated alcoholic picric acid.

Its formation can be inhibited by the use of buffered or neutralized formalin solutions.

Acid fuchsin (acid magenta)

An invaluable histological stain of the phenyl methane family (q.v.), with a wide variety of uses. It is a constituent of Van Gieson's connective tissue stain; it is used for the demonstration of fibrin in the picro-Mallory method, for the demonstration of mitochondria in the Altmann technique, and in several methods of the trichrome group.

Acid fuchsin

Solubility at 20°C is 20.0 per cent in water and 0.25 per cent in alcohol.

Acidophil

Having an affinity for acid dyes, for instance, eosin, acid fuchsin, orange G. The name is applied especially to the alpha cells of the pituitary and of the pancreas.

See also Basophil.

Acid phosphatase

An enzyme found in small amounts in many organs but notably in the prostate, the quantity here being increased at puberty and also in prostatic carcinoma. Its demonstration is based on its ability to hydrolyse sodium glycerophosphate in the presence of lead ions at pH 4.7 with the formation of insoluble lead phosphate at the sites of activity. This is converted to black lead sulphide by the action of ammonium sulphide.

Acridine orange

A fluorochrome related to the xanthene dyes. It has recently found favour in the differential demonstration of DNA and RNA, the former giving a green, and the latter a red/brown fluorescence.

Acridine orange

Acrylic resins

A series of colourless, transparent resins of compact texture, used as infiltration and embedding media in the preparation of very thin sections (500 Å–0.05 μm or less) for electron microscopy.

In histology, the methacrylates, notably n-butyl and methyl $(CH_2:C(CH_3).COO.CH_3)$, are most widely used, often as admixtures in varying proportions with each other and with a plasticiser (such as dibutyl phthalate), and a catalyst (for instance, benzoyl peroxide) which expedites the conversion of the viscous monomeric to the solid polymeric medium essential for ultra-microtomy.

Actinomyces

This fungus may be demonstrated effectively in sections by Gridley's method (a PAS/aldehyde fuchsin combination), the PAS technique itself, or the Gram methods.

Adenosine triphosphatase

A complex phosphomonoesterase found mainly in skeletal and cardiac muscle and in liver. Its demonstration may be effected either by the Wachstein and Meisel technique using a lead-magnesium incubating medium at pH 7.2, or by the Padykula and Herman method with calcium chloride, incubation here being carried out at pH 9.4.

Adhesives

Substances containing albumin, starch, or gelatin, used for attaching tissue sections to slides prior to staining. Only a very small amount of adhesive should be applied and spread evenly on to grease-free slides.

See also Albumin (Mayer's).

Adrenal (suprarenal) gland

The adrenal glands are small asymmetrical flattened bodies, one attached to the upper pole of each kidney. A single gland comprises two distinct organs, cortex and medulla, each with separate functions.

The cortex occupies the greater part of the gland and is composed of three vaguely defined layers: (1) the zona glomerulosa, immediately below the capsule; (2) the zona fasciculata, continuous with and deep to it; and (3) the zona reticularis which is in contact with the central medullary core.

The cortical cells are rich in lipid, mainly cholesterol esters, and in ascorbic acid (vitamin C).

The medullary cells secrete the hormones adrenalin and noradrenalin, which are demonstrable as fine brown granules after oxidation by potassium dichromate. This is known as the 'chromaffin reaction'.

The adrenal cortex is essential to life; its functions are numerous and include maintenance of electrolytic and water balance; it also maintains connective tissues and regulates carbohydrate, protein, and fat metabolism.

The adrenal medulla is not essential to life. The secretion and storage of adrenalin are increased under conditions of physical and emotional stress. This hormone affects blood pressure and clotting-time, carbohydrate metabolism, digestive processes, and so on, in a manner similar to sympathetic nerve stimulation.

Adrenalin

A hormone secreted by the adrenal medulla (q.v.), which may be demonstrated histochemically by (1) the chromaffin techniques using potassium dichromate and subsequent treatment with the Romanovsky group of stains; (2) the Vulpian reaction using ferric chloride; (3) Schmorl's ferric-ferricyanide test; and (4) other methods for reducing substances, including ammoniacal silver solutions.

Adsorption

The property of solid bodies to attract and condense liquid and gaseous substances on to their free surfaces. Supporters of the physical theories of staining have suggested this phenomenon as the likeliest mode of action of stains.

Albumin (Mayer's)

A formula utilizing egg-white mixed with glycerin and water, used as an adhesive (q.v.) for sections.

5

Alcian blue

A basic dye, derived from copper phthalocyanin (CuPC), a stable, water-insoluble, bluish-green compound, rendered soluble by the introduction into the molecule of chloromethyl groups. It is an excellent stain for connective tissue mucins and most epithelial mucins, and is best employed in weak acidified aqueous solution. The reaction may be intensified by prior treatment in chromic or periodic acid. Derivatives of CuPC, such as alcian blue or its alcian green variants, have a considerable advantage over most other mucin stains, because of their great stability and resistance to bleaching or to extraction by subsequent counterstaining procedures.

Solubility at $20°C$ is 5.0 per cent in water and 1.65 per cent in alcohol.

Copper phthalocyanin

Alcohol, ethyl (C_2H_5OH)

A clear, colourless, inflammable fluid; sg 0.798; bp $78.5°C$; miscible with water in all proportions.

Its uses in histology include (1) fixation, alone or in combination, for example, Carnoy's fluid; (2) dehydration of tissues and of sections; (3) manufacture of reagent and stain solutions; (4) differentiation; and (5) restoration of colour to gross specimens for museum demonstration.

Aldehyde

One of a group of substances formed by the oxidation of alcohols, and yielding on further oxidation the fatty acids. It is characterized by the $- C\!\!\begin{smallmatrix} H \\ \\ O \end{smallmatrix}$ group.

Demonstrated histochemically by the Schiff leuco-fuchsin reagent, by phenylhydrazine, by naphthoic acid hydrazide, etc., or negatively demonstrated by various blocking techniques.

Aldolase

An enzyme thought to be involved in the dissimilation of glycogen in muscle. A method of demonstration is based on conversion of hexosediphosphate by the enzyme to triosephosphate, from which phosphates are liberated and precipitated in alkaline solution. These in turn are converted to cobalt phosphate, and finally to brownish-black sulphide by the action of cobalt acetate and ammonium sulphide respectively.

Aliesterases

A group of enzymes comprising the lipases and the non-specific esterases, and forming, together with the cholinesterases, the second main subgroup of enzymes. Differentiation between lipases and non-specific esterases is difficult; but whereas the former are capable of hydrolysing glycerol esters of long-chain fatty acids, the non-specific esterases will attack preferentially the simpler aliphatic esters. Moreover the unsaturated Tweens are hydrolysed by lipases but not by non-specific esterases.

See also Lipase; Cholinesterase; Tweens.

Alimentary tract

The digestive system comprising those organs which are involved in the ingestion and assimilation of food, and the excretion of its waste products. The food enters the mouth, is passed via the pharynx through the oesophagus to the stomach; and thence by way of the duodenum, jejunum, and ileum (which together constitute the small intestine), through the ileocaecal valve, at which point is attached the vermiform appendix; into the caecum, colon, and rectum (forming together the large intestine), and ultimately into the anal canal from which the waste matter (faeces) is expelled through the anal orifice. Associated at various levels with the digestive tract are organs such as the teeth, tongue, and salivary glands; and the liver, gall bladder, and pancreas.

See also Intestine.

Aliphatic compounds

Organic compounds, in which the carbon atoms are arranged in long chains, in contradistinction to the closed-ring arrangement of the aromatic compounds, derived from benzene. The paraffins, fatty acids, and alcohols are examples of aliphatic compounds.

Alizarin

A yellow dye of the anthraquinone group (q.v.). It is employed widely in the demonstration of calcium (especially in the Dawson technique for whole specimens), the skeletal structure being mani-fested as a reddish-purple framework against a transparent background. It is sometimes used in the sulphonated form, which gives a rather more intense colouration.

Alizarin (sulphonated)

Solubility at 20°C is 7.69 per cent in water and 0.15 per cent in alcohol.

Alkaline phosphatase

This enzyme, sometimes referred to as phosphomonoesterase I, is present in most body tissues and fluids; the greatest concentrations are found in actively ossifying cartilage and periosteum, intestinal mucosa, kidney, and liver. Fixation in cold acetone or by freeze-drying is recommended, followed by paraffin or double-embedding. Histochemical identification is based on the principle that, when sections are incubated with sodium glycerophosphate substrate at an alkaline pH in the presence of calcium ions, liberated phosphate ions will be precipitated at the site of formation as insoluble calcium phosphate. These may then be visualized by either of two methods: (1) conversion to black cobalt sulphide, or (2) conversion to silver phosphate and subsequent reduction to metallic silver (von Kóssa's method). Coupling azo dye methods are also available.

Aloxite hone

A bonded or composition stone manufactured in various grades, the finest being eminently suitable for final honing of microtome knives.

Alpha cells

Granular cells of the pancreatic islets or the anterior lobe of the pituitary, normally having a marked affinity for acid dyes such as eosin and orange G, and indeed in the pituitary usually referred to as acidophil cells.

A differential demonstration of alpha and beta cells may be effected with the Masson trichrome group, or with the PAS-orange G method (pituitary) or Gomori's aldehyde fuchsin-orange G-light green (pancreas).

Altmann, Richard (1852–1900)

German histologist, a pioneer of freeze-drying; probably best known for his study of mitochondria and the method, using an aniline-acid fuchsin, which he devised for their demonstration.

Alumina, aluminium oxide (Al_2O_3)
See Abrasive powder.

Alums
A group of double sulphates, employed widely as mordants, notably with haematoxylin. The most important are (1) aluminium potassium sulphate (potassium alum) $Al_2(SO_4)_3.K_2SO_4.24H_2O$, in Ehrlich's haematoxylin; (2) ammonium aluminium sulphate (ammonium alum) $Al_2(SO_4)_3.(NH_4)_2SO_4.24H_2O$ in Delafield's haematoxylin; (3) ammonium ferric sulphate (iron alum) $(NH_4)_2SO_4.Fe_2(SO_4)_3.24H_2O$ in conjunction with Heidenhain's and Loyez haematoxylins; and (4) chromic potassium sulphate (chrome alum) $Cr_2(SO_4)_3.K_2SO_4.24H_2O$ in Gomori's haematoxylin and in Einarson's gallocyanin method for Nissl substance.

Amine
One of a series of compounds produced by the replacement by alkyl radicals of one, two, or three of the hydrogen atoms of ammonia (NH_3), forming primary, secondary, and tertiary amines respectively. Quaternary amines, arising from ammonium hydroxide (NH_4OH), also exist.

Amino acids
A series of very important organic compounds, some twenty or more occurring naturally, containing one or more amino (NH_2) groups in addition to the carboxyl (COOH) group and having the general formula $R - CH - NH_2 - COOH$. From these units the widely diverse protein group is built.

Amino group
The univalent group $-NH_2$, apart from being an essential feature of the amino acids (q.v.), is also of considerable importance in stain chemistry. It is a widely-occurring auxochrome and is present in numerous basic dyes, e.g. in the azures, toluidine blue, and so on, which go to make up the thiazin group.

Amitosis
Simple division of cells which may occur in certain normal and pathological tissues by direct cleavage of the nucleus, there being no evidence of mitotic phases.
See also Mitosis.

Amyloid
Although the precise nature of this substance is obscure it is thought to be a chondroitin sulphuric acid-protein complex.

It is deposited in connective tissue in certain pathological conditions, e.g. as a primary condition not associated with an obvious predisposing disease (primary amyloidosis); or as a sequel to chronic inflammatory conditions such as tuberculosis (secondary amyloidosis).

Amyloid is a homogeneous, translucent substance, so called because it stains similarly to starch (amylos = starch) when treated with iodine. Two of its important features are its metachromatic staining with certain basic dyes and its stainability by iodine, which may be applied to slices of tissue for museum purposes or to sections. It is insoluble in water, alcohol, ether, and weak acids. Other methods for its demonstration include staining with Congo red and impregnation with silver.

Anabolism

Synthetic or constructive metabolism; the assimilation and conversion by chemical action of nutritive material into more complex living matter.

Anaphase

The third stage of mitosis (q.v.).

Anaplasia

A change in the character of a cell, by which it reverts to a more primitive embryonic form, often associated with malignancy.

Ångström unit

A unit of length equivalent to 10^{-10} metre or $1/10,000$ micrometre, devised for the measurement of wave-lengths of all forms of light rays and of intra-molecular distances; currently adopted as the standard in electron-microscopy techniques. Designated by the symbols Å or Å.U.

Aniline ($C_6H_5.NH_2$)

A benzene derivative, poisonous and inflammable, which darkens on exposure to light and air. B.p. $184.4°C$. Its main uses in histology are as a dye solvent, e.g. acid fuchsin in Altmann's technique for mitochondria, and crystal violet and allied stains in the Gram methods for organisms and fibrin, where it may also be mixed with xylene as a differentiating fluid.

Aniline blue WS

The name given to a mixture of phenyl methane dyes, mainly water blue and methyl blue (q.v.), and behaving in identical fashion

10

to these components. It is widely used as a connective tissue and cytoplasmic granule stain in Masson's trichrome method and its variants, but no useful purpose seems to be served in regarding aniline blue WS as a separate entity.

Anisotropic

Certain substances possess the power of rotating polarized light (q.v.) and appear bright against a dark ground. They are described as anisotropic, birefringent, or doubly-refractile.

Common substances having this property include hair and certain lipids, such as myelin, and many inorganic compounds, such as silica and talc.

Antemedium

A term preferred by some workers to denote the various wax, celloidin, or resin solvents used in tissue processing that immediately precedes infiltration in one of these media. Examples of antemedia are the common clearing agents (q.v.), ether-alcohol, methyl benzoate, amyl acetate, and butyl phthalate.

Anthracosis

The deposition of carbon particles in the lungs and associated lymph nodes, arising environmentally or occupationally. In the latter case, e.g. in coal-miners, it can give rise to a form of pneumoconiosis, often in association with silicosis.

See also Carbon.

Anthraquinone dyes

A group of dyes characterized by the inclusion of three linked benzene rings, the central one showing quinoid linkage, thus:

the group includes alizarin and purpurin, both of which may be used in the demonstration of calcium.

Aorta

The main arterial trunk of the body, conveying oxygenated blood from the heart. Its wall is composed largely of dense elastic tissue.

11

Abnormally fatty and calcareous plaques may be found. Processing may effectively be carried out by the 'Swiss roll' method (q.v.).

Applicable staining methods can be found under the appropriate headings, namely Elastic tissue, Lipid, Calcium.

Apáthy's medium

A widely-used aqueous mountant, containing gum arabic and cane sugar, plus a preservative such as thymol. It may be employed in most frozen-section techniques and, because it is not appreciably auto-fluorescent, serves as a valuable mounting medium in fluorescence microscopy. The addition to the mountant of potassium acetate or sodium chloride (Highman's modification) largely inhibits the 'bleeding' of metachromatic stains for amyloid.

Aposiderin

An artefact pigment, formed by the conversion of haemosiderin by acid fixation and giving a negative reaction to Perls' Prussian blue test. It is highly resistant to solution even in strong acids or alkalis, and is not readily bleached. Its superficial similarity to the lipo-fuscins may be discounted by its negative reaction with Schmorl's test for reducing substances.

Appendix vermiform

A blind evagination of the caecum, thick-walled and with a small lumen.

Large amounts of lymphoid tissue are present in the muscular wall; the mucosal epithelium, in which are found crypts of Lieberkühn, is composed of columnar cells, many of them mucus-secreting. Paneth and argentaffin cells also occur.

Aquawax

See Waxes.

Araldite

See Epoxy resins.

Areolar tissue

A loose meshwork of fibrous tissue, comprising collagen and a few elastic fibres with their concomitant cells, commonly called 'loose connective tissue', it connects the skin to the underlying structures, and often forms a link between organs requiring easy alteration in their relative positions.

Argentaffin

Having the innate ability to blacken silver nitrate of its own accord, the reduction taking place as a result of the intrinsic chemical

nature of certain substances, e.g., melanin and ascorbic acid.
See also Argyrophil.

Argentaffin cells (Kultschitsky, enterochromaffin cells)

Isolated granular cells found in the mucosa of the stomach and intestines. They secrete 5-hydroxy-tryptamine which is thought to play a part in muscle contraction and therefore to control, in some measure, peristalsis. Arising from these cells, tumours known as argentaffinoma or carcinoid seem to support this hypothesis. The cell granules are autofluorescent and are capable of reducing silver nitrate and Schmorl's ferric ferricyanide. They may also be demonstrated effectively by a diazonium technique.

Arginine

A strongly basic amino acid essential to life, occurring widely in proteins and forming an important link in nitrogen excretion. It is a constituent of insulin. It may be demonstrated in tissue sections by the Sakaguchi reaction using α-naphthol in conjunction with sodium hypochlorite or hypobromite in alkali, a transitory red colour being produced.

Argyrophil

Possessing an affinity for silver solutions in conjunction with reducing substances such as formalin, hydroquinone, and pyrogallol, whereby a selective deposition of metallic silver occurs on certain specified tissue elements, e.g., reticulin, neurofibrils, glycogen.

Arkansas hone

A hard, pale yellow stone of fine grade, suitable for final honing of microtome knives.

Aromatic compounds

See Aliphatic compounds.

Artefact

A term applied to histological preparations denoting a wide range of aberrant appearances which may be induced by numerous diverse factors: (1) by faulty manipulation; (2) by the physical action of fixative or other reagents; (3) by contamination with extraneous matter. Examples from the first group include most of the cutting artefacts: creases, chatters, compression by a blunt knife; fragmentation of soft tissues during embedding; 'pseudo-emphysema' of lung caused by inexpert use of the vacuum-embedding bath. From the second group: formalin and mercury fixation deposits (*see* Acid formaldehyde haematin and Mercuric chloride); distortion of tissues brought about by processing reagents such as alcohol, xylene, and wax; precipitation of solutions used for staining or for metallic impregnations. In the third group 'knife-carries', i.e. the accidental inclusion of a fragment of foreign tissue; the deposition of squamous epithelial cells caused by 'huffing' on the paraffin block during section-cutting; and generally the introduction of various foreign bodies such as dust, textile fibres, hairs, etc. Also of an artefactual nature is the false localization of tissue substances such as enzymes, pigments, and lipids induced either by faulty manipulation or by the agency of the solutions employed.

Asbestos (fibrous magnesium and calcium silicate)

Asbestos pneumoconiosis (asbestosis) is a lung disease which occurs in asbestos workers owing to inhalation of asbestos fibres. In these cases highly characteristic asbestos bodies may be found microscopically in the sputum and lungs and (rarely) in the associated lymph nodes. The bodies are composed of a central asbestos fibre covered by an iron-protein substance. They are golden-yellow segmented structures with bulbous ends, varying in shape and size, remaining permanently in situ, and are never phagocytozed. They give a powerful Prussian blue reaction for ferric iron.

Astrocytes (astroglia)

The predominant variety of neuroglial cells, they are of two types: (1) protoplasmic astrocytes, found chiefly in the grey matter and possessing a large nucleus, abundant granular cytoplasm with thick branching processes, and containing no visible fibres; and (2) fibrous or fibrillary astrocytes, more abundant in the white matter and distinguished from (1) by their long, thin, smooth, rarely-branching processes and having within the cytoplasm fibrillary structures (neuroglia fibres). Both types may be attached to blood vessels by elongated processes known as sucker feet or footplates. Methods for their demonstration include the metallic impregnations of Cajal, Hortega, and Scharenberg, and the methods of Mallory, Holzer, and Anderson.

Atrophy

The wasting or shrinkage of an organ or of its constituent tissues or cells as a result of malnutrition of physiological or pathological origin. It is often accompanied by some degree of degeneration or even necrosis.

Auramine

A fluorochrome of the phenyl methane group, used alone, or in conjunction with rhodamine for the demonstration of *Mycobacterium tuberculosis,* which gives a yellow fluorescence.

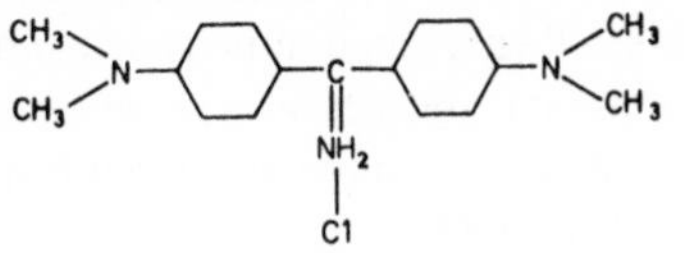

Auramine

Aurantia

A yellow dye of the nitro-series, used in the Champy-Kull mitochondria technique.

It is highly toxic, inducing a troublesome dermatitis.

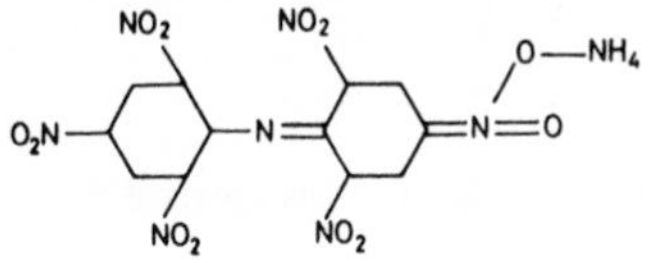

Aurantia

Autolysis

Lysis or destruction of cells by intracellular proteolytic enzyme action following cell death. Autolysis may be retarded by low temperatures and arrested by fixation.

See also Cathepsins and Lysosome.

Autoradiography (ARG)

Techniques whereby the presence of radioactive isotopes in tissues may be determined, the principle being the exposure of photographic emulsion to a tissue section containing an isotope, long enough to allow the radioactivity to reduce the silver in the emulsion. After development the reduced silver is visible as black granules. Distribution, and an approximate quantitative estimation of radioactivity in cells and tissues may thus be determined.

Auxochrome

A chemical group, e.g., the OH (hydroxyl) or NH_2 (amino) radicles, whose presence confers upon a coloured benzene derivative (a chromogen) the properties of a true dye. It is responsible for the dye's power of retention, preventing its ready extraction, and determines in large measure its acid or basic nature.

See also Chromophore.

Axon (axis cylinder)

That cytoplasmic process of a nerve cell (neurone) which transmits excitation or nervous impulses from the cell to an effector

15

organ. Usually thinner and much longer than the dendrites of the same cell, the axon is a fine thread of fairly uniform thickness, which does not branch freely until it approaches its termination (axon ending). The axon of a nerve cell enveloped in its neurilemmal and medullary sheaths (where present), constitutes a nerve fibre. Methods for their demonstration are based on ammoniacal silver impregnation typified by the Bielschowsky technique.

Azins

A family of dyes having as their chromophoric group two benzene rings, one showing quinoid arrangement, linked by two nitrogen atoms, thus:

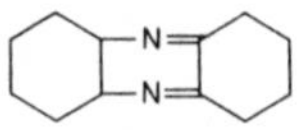

It includes such useful red basic dyes as neutral red, safranin, and azocarmine.

Azocarmine

A red basic dye of the azin group (q.v.) commonly employed in conjunction with aniline blue WS as an alternative to Masson's trichrome stain, and perhaps preferable to it on certain tissues, notably kidney.

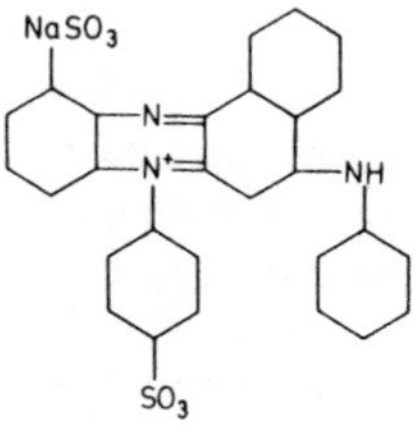

Azocarmine G

Azo dyes

A group of dyes characterized by the presence of two linked chromophoric nitrogen atoms between paired benzene or naph-thalene rings. This configuration may be single, as in the mono-azo subgroup:

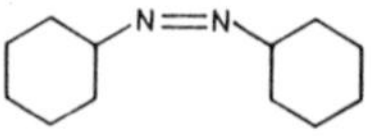

Mono-azo

or double or even multiple, as in the disazo and polyazo subgroups, e.g., the disazo:

16

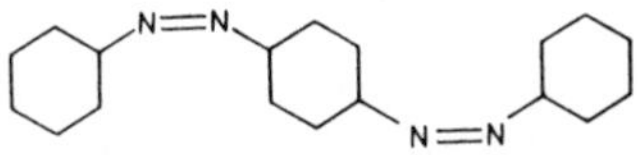

Disazo

Among the mono-azo dyes in common use are Orange G, Janus green, and Metanil yellow; whilst of the disazo and polyazo dyes, the fat-soluble Sudan stains, Biebrich scarlet, Bismarck brown, Congo red, and Trypan blue are probably the best known.

Azures

A range of blue dyes of the thiazin group, and labelled A, B, and C according to the number of CH_3 (methyl) groups attached to the thionin molecule, and intermediate between it and methylene blue which upon oxidation or 'polychroming' is partially converted to them. When added to eosin, aqueous solutions of these dyes form precipitates which are insoluble in water, but readily soluble in alcohol to form the so-called 'neutral stains'. These constitute the basis of the Romanovsky dyes, so widely used in haematological methods such as Leishman and Giemsa.

B

Bacteria

In the wide sense, all micro-organisms, with the exception at the one extreme of the algae and protozoa, and at the other of the viruses.

See also Micro-organisms.

Balsam, Canada

A natural resin soluble in xylene, toluene, or chloroform, at one time almost universally employed as a mounting medium (R.I. 1.52) for sections. It has tended in recent years to be replaced by plastic mountants such as the polystyrenes, perhaps regrettably, as there is evidence that stain preservation over a long period is superior in balsam-mounted sections, particularly those stained with haematoxylin and eosin.

Basement membrane

The delicate, noncellular, transparent layer underlying the epithelium of mucous membranes and secreting glands. Its demonstration, notably in the kidney, can be effected by the PAS and the Masson trichrome methods.

17

Basic dye

A stain compound in which the colouring property is in the basic component, this property being imparted by the contained basic chromophoric and auxochromic groups. Such dyes are salts of a colour base, often chloride, sometimes acetate or sulphate, and normally have an affinity for the more acidic tissue elements.

The common basic dyes include methylene blue, neutral red, gallocyanin, basic fuchsin.

See also Acid dye.

Basic fuchsin

A basic stain, or more often, a mixture of stains of the phenyl methane group with a wide diversity of uses in histology, the most important of which are (1) in Weigert's resorcin-fuchsin mixture for elastic fibres; (2) in Macchiavello's technique for Rickettsia and various inclusion bodies; (3) in the Ziehl-Neelsen method for acid-fast bacilli; (4) in Gomori's aldehyde fuchsin method for elastic tissue and for cells of the pancreas and pituitary; and (5) as the main constituent in Schiff's reagent for the detection of aldehydes.

The stain as a rule is supplied commercially as mixtures of triamino-triphenyl methanes with one, two, or three methyl (CH_3) groups present

Solubility at $20°C$ is 0.26 per cent in water and 5.93 per cent in alcohol.

Basic fuchsin

Basophil

In histology, a term applied to any tissue constituent possessing an affinity for basic dyes, such as haematoxylin, methylene blue, and basic fuchsin. The reaction of such tissue components is normally acidic, examples including chromatin, mast cell granules, and some mucins.

Beeswax

A mixture of fatty acid esters obtained from the honeycomb. It is a yellowish substance (mp $60°C$–$65°C$), miscible with paraffin wax and the fat solvents. Admixtures with paraffin wax are used to obtain a harder, more consistent, somewhat 'stickier' medium, well-suited to serial sectioning techniques.

Belgian hone

A yellow stone, very popular for routine microtome knife sharpening, and with a reasonably fast action.

Benign

A term applied to diseases in general, but with particular reference to neoplasms or new-growths, and implying a comparatively innocent nature favouring recovery.

See also Malignant.

Benzene (C_6H_6)

The most important of the hydrocarbons. Its generally accepted formula is:

usually abbreviated to   *Benzene*

It is poisonous and highly inflammable and, although up till recently it was widely employed as a clearing agent, its highly carcinogenic nature would strongly discourage its further use in this field. It is the parent substance upon which the manufacture of the synthetic dyes is based.

Benzidine ($C_{12}H_{12}N_2$)

A noxious compound (it is a powerful carcinogen) still occasionally used for the detection of haemoglobin (Lepehne's method). The benzidine is oxidized by the peroxidase-peroxide system to form a brown or blue compound. The method has been largely superseded by the Lison-Dunn leuco-patent blue method.

Benzoylation

A blocking procedure rendering hydroxyl and amine groupings nonreactive. Treatment of glycogen, for example, for six hours at $58°C$ with a mixture of benzoyl chloride and anhydrous pyridine completely destroys its reactivity. Washing in descending concentrations of alcohol (100 per cent, 95 per cent, 80 per cent) should follow the benzoylation.

See also Blocking.

Beryllium

Compounds of this element are occasionally encountered in

19

tissues as the result of occupational hazards; they are extremely toxic. Demonstration of beryllium may be effected by naphthochrome green B, using acridine red as a counterstain (Denz's method).

Beta cells

Granular cells of the pancreatic islets or of the anterior lobe of the pituitary. The former are stained well by the Gomori aldehyde fuchsin method, the latter by Schiff's reagent. Both types of cell are stained by aniline blue or light green in the Masson trichrome techniques.

Bevels, stropping

More accurately called knife-backs, they are tubular devices fitted on to the backs of microtome knives during honing and stropping. By this means the back of the knife is raised by a constant amount, thus imparting the necessary bevel to the knife-edge.

Biebrich scarlet

An acid dye of the disazo family, sometimes employed in the trichrome methods in place of acid fuchsin.

Biebrich scarlet

Bielschowsky, Max (1869–1940)

A German neuropathologist and, in company with his Spanish contemporary, Ramón y Cajal, one of the great pioneers of the metallic impregnation methods. His technique for the demonstration of neurofibrils is employed universally and is the basis for countless modifications.

Bile canaliculi

These are intercellular channels running between liver cells, frequently anastomozing with one another. They may be well demonstrated with Mallory's phosphotungstic acid haematoxylin and also by some metallic impregnations.

Bile pigments

These are extracellular pigments arising from haemoglobin breakdown and known alternatively as haematoidin; they are found especially in foci of old haemorrhage and in infarcts. The pigments exist essentially in two forms: bilirubin, ranging in colour from lemon yellow to reddish-brown crystals or amorphous masses; and biliverdin, a greenish pigment which is the oxidized form of bilirubin, and is found characteristically in the liver and gall-bladder. The least oxidized form, that is, the lemon-yellow bilirubin, may be demonstrated histologically by the Gmelin test using nitric acid (about 50 per cent — the reaction with concentrated acid is much too rapid for critical observation). A colour change takes place ranging through green, blue, purple, red, and pink, the pigment finally dissolving. Bilirubin has been shown to contain a powerful reducing substance, and in consequence gives strongly positive Schmorl and Fontana reactions. This property decreases as the degree of oxidation of the pigment increases, negative reactions occurring with hepatic biliverdin. Stein's iodine method is sometimes used, but its value is limited, inasmuch as a positive reaction is only obtained with partially oxidized forms of bilirubin.

Bilirubin Biliverdin
See Bile pigments.

Birefringence (or double refraction)
The property possessed by certain substances of splitting a single incident ray of light into two emergent rays at right angles to each other. Examples of birefringent (or anisotropic) material include hair, talc, starch, collagen, and some lipids.
See also Polaroid; Nicol prisms; Polarization of light.

Bismarck brown
A basic dye of the disazo family, a constituent of the Papanicolaou cytological stain and occasionally employed as a stain for mucin.

Bismarck brown

Heating should be avoided when preparing solutions of Bismarck brown as this dye is unstable.
Solubility at $20°C$ is 1.0 per cent in water and 1.0 per cent in alcohol.

Bismuth
Compounds of this element may occasionally be found in tissues. Their demonstration may be effected by Wachstein and Zak's method, using brucine or quinine sulphate and potassium iodide, whereupon an orange-red iodobismuthate is obtained.

Bladder
The urinary bladder is a sac situated in the anterior part of the

pelvis, to which urine is passed by the ureters from the kidneys, and from which, by means of the urethra, it is excreted. Its wall is composed largely of involuntary muscle and it is lined by transitional epithelium.

Bleaching

(1) A procedure used for the differential diagnosis of pigments in tissues; for example, the decolourization of melanin by chlorine or potassium permanganate and oxalic acid (the Mallory bleach).

(2) The whitening of bones, for example, by hydrogen peroxide, after removal of the soft tissues by maceration and prior to mounting as a museum specimen.

Block impregnation

A technique whereby certain tissue elements or inclusions may be treated with some metallic salt or salts before processing and embedding. Some tissue components, notably Golgi apparatus and nerve endings, and some organisms, spirochaetes for example, lend themselves to such techniques. With these, a more uniform and reliable demonstration is possible than with methods that entail the more orthodox impregnation on the slide.

Blocking

This, in histological technique, has two quite distinct meanings.

(1)   In processing it is used to denote the embedding or casting of the tissue in paraffin wax or some other medium.

(2)   In histochemistry, a blocking or blockade technique is a chemical procedure which, although it fails to give a colour reaction with a certain tissue element, will combine with that element so as to preclude it from reacting with some other agent. Benzoylation and acetylation are examples of such techniques (q.v.).

Blood pigments

Pigments derived from blood include acid-formaldehyde haematin, the haemosiderins, aposiderin, malarial pigment (haemozoin), haemoglobin, and bile pigments, and may be found under these headings.

See also Pigments, haematogenous.

Bone

A hard form of connective tissue containing specialized cells known as osteocytes, and a calcified collagenous material often arranged in thin layers known as lamellae. Its constituent cells derive their nutriment from tissue fluids originating from the capillary blood and diffusing through minute canals (canaliculi) which permeate the bony matrix. These tiny spaces are produced by the bone-forming cells (osteoblasts) which secrete the organic intercellular substance of the bone and possess long cytoplasmic processes; these processes link up with adjacent osteoblasts and, when the material so formed hardens, they disintegrate, leaving the canaliculi in their place. Some osteoblasts proliferate along the margins of the bone they have formed, others surround themselves with the secreted material to become osteocytes. Bone may occur in two forms: (1) spongy or cancellous bone, consisting of a delicate framework of spidery processes or spicules (spicules radiate from an ossification centre and join up to form an elaborate scaffolding of trabeculae); and (2) compact or ivory bone which is made up of large numbers of Haversian systems.

The Haversian system may be regarded as the unit of compact bone structure; it consists of a series of lamellae, usually arranged concentrically around a narrow lumen containing one or two blood-vessels. The lamellae possess numerous small spaces called lacunae communicating with each other and with the central lumen by means of the canaliculi, each lacuna containing an osteocyte. Over-proliferation of the bone is controlled by the presence of osteoclasts, large multinucleate cells whose mode of action probably resembles that of foreign-body giant cells and which produce an enzyme that dissolves the cement substance of the bone matrix. Although sections of undecalcified bone may be obtained by some modern techniques, it is customary to remove the calcium salts (decalcification, q.v.) prior to embedding in paraffin wax or celloidin. Sectioning is thus considerably facilitated. Staining methods applicable to bone sections, apart from haematoxylin and eosin, include Schmorl's techniques for bone canaliculi, and the general connective tissue methods.

Borax-ferricyanide

Solutions containing sodium tetraborate and potassium ferricyanide may be employed as bleaching or differentiating fluids. Melanin and the silver complex of argyria may be so bleached. As a differentiator it may be used following haematoxylin in Loyez' method for myelin sheaths, and in Baker's acid haematein method for phospholipids, among others.

Bordeaux red

An acid dye of the mono-azo group, sometimes used as a counterstain to haematoxylin or as an alternative to ponceau de xylidine in the Masson techniques.

Bordeaux red

Solubility at 20°C is 3.8 per cent in water and 0.19 per cent in alcohol.

Bouin, Paul (1870–1962)

A French anatomist, whose fixative, devised in 1897, is employed routinely in some laboratories, most widely in his native country. It contains picric acid, formalin, and acetic acid, and may be used not only as a micro-anatomical but also often as a cytological fixative. It is especially suitable in view of its picric acid content for glycogen preservation.

Boutons terminaux

The small button-like discs which constitute the synaptic endings of some nerve fibres. The boutons terminaux are in contact with the dendrites or cell bodies of neurones remote from the cell of origin of the nerve fibres which bear them.

Brain

The mass of nervous material within the cranium, including the cerebrum, the cerebellum, and the brain stem. In conjunction with the spinal cord it constitutes the central nervous system (CNS). The cerebrum comprises two hemispheres, joined by the corpus callosum, each consisting of a superficial layer of grey matter (cortex), and a deep mass of white matter (medulla), composed largely of myelinated fibres. The cerebellum (hind-brain) has a somewhat similar structure, insofar as it is invested with a thin grey cortical layer, but histologically its component cells differ markedly from those of the cerebrum. The brain stem which merges at its lower margin with the spinal cord consists of an intimate admixture of grey and white matter.

A wide range of techniques has been devised for the demonstration, often selective, of the various cells and their fibrillary processes.

The most important techniques are dealt with under their respective headings.

See Astrocytes; Oligodendroglia; Microglia; Neurones; Neurofibrils; Axons; Nerve endings; Nissl bodies; Myelin.

Brazilin

A natural basic dye, analogous to haematoxylin, and oxidizing in similar fashion to form brazilein, the active stain component. As

with haematoxylin, mordanting with alum or ferric salts is necessary.
The probable formula for brazilein is:

Brazilein

Bromination

A system of blocking techniques (*see also* acetylation and
methylation) whereby the demonstration of certain chemical groups
is inhibited. The ethylenic group $-C = C-$, for example, to be found
in unsaturated lipids and in certain lipofuscin-type pigments, may
normally be demonstrated by Schiff's reagent following oxidation
in performic acid (PFAS) or peracetic acid (PAAS). Mode of fixation
and sectioning is influenced by the solubility requirements of the
substance under study. Pretreatment, however, with bromine, either
in aqueous solution (in the case of the soluble lipids) or in carbon
tetrachloride (in the case of lipofuscins) completely blocks these
reactions.

See also Blocking.

Bromuration

The treatment of tissue sections with solutions containing
bromine or one of its compounds. In some neurohistological
techniques, for example, fixation in formalin-ammonium bromide
is advocated or, alternatively, treatment of the cut frozen sections
with hydrobromic acid as a prelude to a metallic impregnation.

'Brown atrophy' pigment

A form of lipofuscin (q.v.) found in heart muscle, known sometimes as 'wear and tear' pigment or Abnützungspigment; it gives a
positive reaction to Sudan black but a negative one to Schmorl's
reagent.

Buffer

A mixture of certain acidic and basic compounds which, when
added to a solution, helps to stabilize its hydrogen-ion concentration (pH) and maintain this at a constant level in spite of the
addition of relatively large amounts of acid or alkali. Such mixtures
are usually combinations either of a weak acid and its salt with a
strong base, or a weak base and its salt with a strong acid. Buffers
are used widely in numerous histochemical techniques, notably in
methods for the demonstration of enzymes and pigments.

C

Cadmium
Salts of cadmium (chloride or nitrate) inhibit the solution of lipids, and hence are often incorporated in fixative mixtures to give optimum preservation. Baker's formalin-cadmium-calcium mixtures and Aoyama's method for Golgi apparatus are examples of this property.

Cajal, Santiago Ramón y (1852–1934)
An illustrious Spanish histologist who, in company with his friend and pupil, del Río Hortega (q.v.), was responsible for most of our knowledge of the micro-anatomy of the nervous system. A brilliant theoretician and technologist, he devised numerous methods, most of them based on metallic impregnation, designed to demonstrate the constituent elements of the nervous tissues; probably the best known of these is his gold chloride-sublimate method for astrocytes (q.v.).

Cajuput oil
A colourless or greenish essential oil with an agreeable odour, used occasionally as a clearing agent for tissues and for celloidin sections. It is also called for as an ingredient, together with creosote, alcohol, and xylene, of Gothard's differentiator in toluidine blue or thionin methods for Nissl substance.

Calcium
Methods of the demonstration of calcium salts in tissue sections may be divided into two main groups: those which indicate the presence of calcium itself, and those which are applicable to phosphates or carbonates in combination with calcium. In the first category and usually present in soluble form, calcium may be demonstrated by precipitation with oxalic or tartaric acids, the insoluble oxalate or tartrate being formed; or by Crétin's method using gallic acid-metaldehyde. Calcium in the form of phosphate or carbonate may be identified by impregnation with silver nitrate (von Kóssa) or by the formation of calcium lakes with dyes of the anthraquinone group such as purpurin or alizarin. This last named dye is also employed in Dawson's technique for the skeletal structure of mammalian embryos. Methods for the removal of calcium salts from tissue are dealt with under Decalcification.

Canada balsam
See Balsam, Canada.

Canaliculi (L. dim of *canalis,* a channel)

Small channels to be seen in certain tissues notably in bone and liver.

See also Bile canaliculi; Bone.

Carbohydrate

One of many organic compounds composed of carbon, hydrogen, and oxygen molecules only, and including aldehydes, ketones, and mono- and poly-saccharides. In histochemistry substances such as amyloid, glycogen, and the mucins are notable examples.

Carbon

Commonly classified as an exogenous 'pigment', carbon is found in the lungs, either in macrophages or extracellularly, and in the associated lymph nodes; the quantity varies according to environment, occupation, and age. Its pathological significance is usually negligible, but in large amounts it can give rise to anthracosis, especially in coal miners. It is recognized, apart from its location, by its jet black colour and its resistance to bleaching and solvent action.

Carborundum (silicon carbon, SiC)

A substance of a hardness second only to that of the diamond, it is used as an abrasive in the manufacture of hones; in paste form it is used as a dressing for strops.

Carmine

The aluminium lake of the pigment obtained from the dried females of the cochineal insect, and in fact the only common dye substance to be derived from animal sources. Its value, though largely historic, is still quite considerable; it may be employed either in acid or alkaline solution and behaves accordingly as a basic or acidic dye. Its active principle is carminic acid.

Carminic acid

Mordanting with metallic compounds (of aluminium, magnesium, or iron) is necessary, and among its uses are the demonstration of glycogen (Best's method) and mucin (Southgate's and Mayer's methods). It is occasionally called for as a red nuclear stain (followed by an aqueous mountant) as a counterstain, for example, to Sudan Black B.

Carnoy's fluid

A fixative containing alcohol, chloroform, and acetic acid, widely used by virtue of its rapid action for routine, especially urgent, biopsy material. It is a valuable cytological (nuclear) fixative.

Carotenoids

A group of exogenous pigments, derivatives of carotene ($C_{40}H_{56}$), and occurring naturally on a very wide scale. They are red to yellow in colour and are responsible for colouring such vegetables as carrots and swedes, and in the animal kingdom for bird plumage and the brilliant hue of goldfish etc. The colour of animal fats (e.g., butter, cheese and human adipose tissue) is also due to carotenoid pigments. Two other groups of natural pigments, the chlorophylls and the xanthophylls, are closely related to the carotenoids, the colouration of corpora lutea, adrenal cortex, and egg yolk being due to pigments of the xanthophyll group. Such exogenous pigments are assimilated by dietary means and are elaborated by the liver to form vitamin A. Their demonstration histologically is extremely difficult; they are alleged to yield a transient blue colour with sulphuric acid and a deep violet with iodine, but permanent visualization seems virtually impossible; they exhibit, however, a green fluorescence in ultra-violet light.

Carotid body

A small epithelioid body lying in the bifurcation of the common carotid artery, whose function is now established as a chemoreceptor; its abundant nerve endings respond to chemical changes in the blood, and stimuli are transmitted to those centres in the brain that control the circulatory system.

Cartilage

A special form of connective tissue which is firm, flexible, and slightly elastic; it comprises characteristic cells (chondrocytes) enclosed in a collagenous and mucoid matrix, which exists in the form of a firm gel and possesses a translucent appearance. This typical form is known as hyaline cartilage; an increase in the proportion of collagen fibres, or the presence of elastic fibres transforms it into white fibrocartilage and yellow elastic cartilage respectively. The first type (hyaline cartilage) covers the articular ends of bones in movable joints. The second (fibrocartilage) is found at the sites of tendon insertions and also forms the intervertebral discs. The third type (elastic cartilage) occurs in mobile sites, such as the pinna of the ear and the epiglottis.

Cathepsins

Proteolytic enzymes liberated within the dead cell, causing its ultimate digestion. These enzymes are responsible for the process known as autolysis (q.v.).

Cedarwood oil

A colourless or slightly yellow, somewhat viscid, volatile oil, miscible with alcohol and ether and insoluble in water. It is used as a clearing agent, possessing a slow but gentle action eminently suited to delicate tissues, but has a disadvantage in that it is difficult to eliminate in the paraffin oven.

Celestin blue

A quinone-imine dye of the oxazin subgroup. Now firmly established as a reliable nuclear stain, it has tended to replace or at least to augment haematoxylin staining for certain purposes, notably in the PAS techniques and in the Van Gieson and trichrome methods. Iron alum is normally incorporated in the stain solution as a mordant.

Celestin blue

Celloidin

A form of pyroxylin consisting mainly of cellulose nitrate (nitrocellulose, $C_{12}H_{16}N_4O_{18}$). It is used widely as an embedding medium, notably for bones, eyes, and nervous tissues; it possesses certain advantages over paraffin wax, in that processing can be carried out at room temperature, thus minimizing shrinkage and distortion; greater support is offered to denser tissues and to those of varied consistence, like bone and eye tissues. Because of its explosive nature it is supplied moistened with water or alcohol. For embedding purposes it is customarily dissolved at increasing concentrations in alcohol-ether mixture or in methyl benzoate. It may also be used in conjunction with paraffin wax in the double-embedding technique (q.v.). It is also used in the form of a dilute solution in alcohol-ether for covering cut paraffin or frozen sections prior to staining, as this prevents their detachment from the slides and preserves some diffusible tissue inclusion such as glycogen. Nitrocelluloses of lower viscosity (LVN) (q.v.) are sometimes used as an alternative to celloidin, because of their superior powers of penetration, especially in higher concentrations; harder blocks may thus be obtained, resulting in thinner sections.

Cellosolve

The popular name for 2-ethoxyethanol or ethylene glycol

29

monoethyl ether; it is miscible with water, alcohol, ether, and acetone, is a solvent of paraffin and other waxes, and may be used therefore as both dehydrating and clearing agent. It is occasionally used as a stain solvent, notably for tartrazine in the phloxine-tartrazine sequences.

Centrioles

Cytoplasmic organelles consisting of a pair of small cylindrical bodies situated within the centrosome (q.v.). They are thought to play a part in the organization of fibrillar material such as the cilia, which extend from certain cells, and the astral rays of the achromatic spindle, upon which the chromosomes arrange themselves during mitosis.

Centrosome

A cytoplasmic organelle, known also as the cell centre or attraction sphere. It is an area of condensed protoplasm lying close to the nucleus and is present in most cells. In iron haematoxylin-stained sections it may be seen to contain one or two small dark spheres which are the centrioles (q.v.).

Cephalin

One of the two main types of phosphatides or phospholipids (the other being lecithin, with which it is invariably associated in the tissues); it is distinguished from lecithin by the presence of amino-ethyl alcohol (ethanolamine) as the nitrogenous base in place of choline:

$$H\diagdown_{\underset{\underset{H}{|}}{N}}\diagup CH_2CH_2OH$$

See also Phospholipids.

Cerebrosides

See Galactolipids.

Ceresin

A complex mixture of hydrocarbons, occurring as natural mineral deposits (mp $61°-78°C$). Like beeswax (q.v.), it may be incorporated in paraffin wax for infiltration and embedding purposes to reduce crystallinity, giving a medium with improved sectioning and ribboning properties.

Ceroid

A name given to a fatty pigment or group of pigments of a highly controversial nature; it may occur naturally or be induced experimentally, and is alleged by some authorities to result from vitamin E deficiency. Its separate identity has not been established conclusively and recent work indicates that it is a lipofuscin in an early stage of oxidation. Its reactions (basophilia, acid-fastness, sudanophilia) support this view.

Charcoal, activated

An amorphous, quasi-graphitic form of carbon in the form of small particles. Its main histological application is the removal of the residual colour from Schiff's reagent (q.v.). A method has also been devised for the study of the circulation of the liver using charcoal suspended in gelatin as an injection medium.

Chelation

The ability of certain compounds to form a ring structure of atoms enclosing a central, usually metallic, ion. Haemoglobin and chlorophyll are chelates with an enclosed iron and magnesium atom respectively. Histologically, chelation is utilized as a method of decalcification, calcium ions being bound by, for example, ethylene diamine tetra-acetic acid (EDTA).

Chitin

A horny substance, similar to cellulose, found in the carapaces of crustacea and also in insects, bacteria, protozoa and so on. It is extremely difficult to section but may be softened by treatment with weak acids (a mixture of picric, chromic, and nitric acids is recommended); double embedding (q.v.) is also advocated. Chitin gives a positive reaction to the periodic acid- and chromic acid-Schiff techniques.

Chloral hydrate ($CCl_3.CHO.H_2O$)

A narcotic sometimes used as an accelerator in neuropathological techniques for the demonstration of nerve-endings and neurofibrils by metallic impregnation. It is commonly incorporated in the fixative. It finds occasional use as a preservative in stain solutions such as Mayer's haemalum.

Chloroform ($CHCl_3$)

A heavy, non-inflammable, volatile, colourless liquid widely used as a 'clearing agent' (q.v.) for tissues. Its action is reasonably gentle and fairly slow, and it may be eliminated without great difficulty in the paraffin wax bath; it is therefore to be recommended when extreme rapidity is not called for. Apart from its uses as a clearing agent, it is an ingredient of the popular rapid fixative, Carnoy's fluid (q.v.), and it is also employed in Holzer's neuroglia method as a stain solvent for crystal violet and, together with aniline, as a differentiator.

Chlorophyll

A porphyrin derivative, related to haemoglobin but containing a magnesium instead of a ferric atom, responsible for the green colouration of plants. It may occur as chlorophyll A ($C_{55}H_{72}MgN_4O_5$), bluish-green in colour, or as the oxidized yellowish chlorophyll B ($C_{55}H_{70}MgN_4O_6$). Latterly chlorophyll has found favour as a fluorchrome for the demonstration of neutral lipids, which exhibit a brilliant red fluorescence. It may be used in conjunction with berberine sulphate which imparts to nuclei a contrasting yellow fluorescence.

Cholesterol ($C_{27}H_{45}OH$)

The most important of the sterols and a universal constituent lipid of all mammalian cells. It is especially abundant in nervous tissue and the adrenals, and pathologically in gallstones and atheromatous arteries. It may exist in the free state in the form of characteristic notched rhomboid plates, but is often to be found in ester form which, in the fresh unfixed state, may show a Maltese-cross birefringency. Fixation however induces the formation of acicular crystals. Methods for the demonstration of cholesterol in histological preparations include the Liebermann-Burchardt reaction, the Windaus digitonin method, and the bismuth trichloride technique.

Choline

See Phospholipids.

Cholinesterase

The name given to a group of enzymes by virtue of their ability to hydrolyse esters of choline. They may be divided into two types: acetyl (or true, or specific) cholinesterases and pseudo- (or non-specific) cholinesterases. The former group is associated particularly with the nervous tissue and red blood corpuscles, the motor end-plates in muscle especially showing a high concentration. The pseudo-cholinesterases are found in appreciable amounts in pancreas, salivary, and other glands and also in the blood-serum. Demonstration may be carried out using acetylthiocholine in conjunction with copper sulphate as a substrate, the thiocholine liberated by both acetyl and pseudo-cholinesterases reacting with the copper sulphate to form copper thiocholine. When treated with ammonium sulphide this compound is converted to dark-brown amorphous copper sulphide, which is thus visualized at the sites of activity. Differentiation between acetyl and pseudo-cholinesterases may be effected by the use of a weak solution of di-isopropylfluorophosphate; the pseudo-cholinesterases are thus inhibited and the acetyl compounds remain unimpaired. The pseudo-cholinesterases alone may be shown by the substitution of butyrylthiocholine for acetylthiocholine in the afore-mentioned substrate.

Chromaffin

A term given to certain cells of the adrenal medulla which, when fixed in dichromate solutions, exhibit a dark-brown granular appearance due to the presence of adrenalin (chromaffin reaction). Tissue must be fresh and is best fixed in a formal-dichromate solution such as Régaud's or formal-Muller. Sublimate-containing chrome fixatives such as Helly and Zenker give less constant results, and those containing chromic acid tend to give a negative reaction. It should be stressed that the granules cannot be demonstrated by post-chroming after initial formalin fixation. Apart from the adrenal medulla, chromaffin tissue may be found in the paraganglia, and the reaction is also given by the argentaffin or enterochromaffin cells (q.v.) of the intestine. Unstained sections may be used, but it is customary to employ either toluidine blue or Giemsa's method following the dichromate fixation; in each case the chromaffin cells appear green. The chromaffin reaction is not entirely specific for adrenalin.

See also Vulpian reaction.

Chromatin

A term given to those nuclear aggregations that have an affinity for basic dyes, such as haematoxylin.

Chrome-osmium

The name applied to a group of fixatives containing osmium tetroxide plus chromic acid and/or potassium dichromate.

Chromic acid ($H_2 CrO_4$)

The aqueous solution of the dark red crystalline chromium trioxide (CrO_3). The crystals are deliquescent and highly combustible with most organic solvents. Chromic acid is a fixing agent and is seldom used alone; because of its powerful oxidant properties it is incompatible with either alcohol or formalin. Its main applications as a fixative are in association with osmium tetroxide, for example in Flemming's and Champy's fluids, both of which are excellent cytological fixatives. It is essential that material should be thoroughly washed after such fixation in order to prevent the formation in the tissues of the insoluble chromium oxide ($Cr_2 O_3$), formed by the interaction of alcohol and chromic acid.

Chromic acid is also used, usually in conjunction with sulphuric acid, for cleaning glassware. This mixture should obviously be handled with great respect!

Chromidial substance

See Nissl bodies.

Chromogen

A term used to denote a benzene derivative that is coloured, by virtue of the presence of a chromophoric group, but lacks the auxochrome that would convert it into a dye.

See Chromophore; Auxochrome.

Chromophil

A loose term often applied to intracellular granules, signifying an affinity for stains, and having particular reference to the acidophil and basophil cells of the pituitary.

See Chromophobe.

Chromophobe

Having an aversion to staining. The term is used to describe especially those cells of the pituitary which remain relatively unstained in the trichrome methods, in contradistinction to the chromophil cells, acidophil and basophil.

Chromophore

One of several groups of atoms that may impart to a benzene derivative its coloured properties, the compound thus arising being termed a chromogen. Some chromophores have a basic, others an acidic character. Of the former, the most important are the azo, azin, and quinone-imine groups; and of the latter, the quinone and nitro groups. Each of these is dealt with under the appropriate heading.

See also Auxochrome.

Chromosomes

Small thread-like bodies, common to all living cells, that may be demonstrated during cell division by virtue of their great affinity for basic dyes. The number of chromosomes in all body cells of any given species is, with rare exceptions, fixed and immutable, but varies from one species to another. In man there are 23 pairs of chromosomes, of which one pair are sex chromosomes, similar in the female (XX), dissimilar in the male (XY). Arranged in linear fashion along the chromosomes are concentrations of desoxyribonucleic acid (DNA). These form the physical basis for genes (q.v.), which are responsible for the transmission of hereditary characteristics. Each chromosome has a bifid structure formed by two chromatids lying side by side and linked at one point (the centromere); the two constituent chromatids have identical genetic structure. These chromosomal features are best studied during the

metaphase stage of mitosis, and for this purpose such methods as
Feulgen, Heidenhain's iron alum-haematoxylin, and Unna-
Pappenheim's methyl green-pyronin are probably the most popular.
For squash preparations, acidified orcein or carmine are also used.
See also Sex chromatin; Meiosis; Mitosis.

Chromotrope 2R

An acid mono-azo dye, used occasionally as a substitute for
eosin or for ponceau 2R (*ponceau de xylidine*), especially for the
demonstration of eosinophil leucocytes in tissue sections.

Chromotrope 2R

Solubility at $20°C$ is 19.3 per cent in water and 0.17 per cent in
alcohol.

Clearing agent

A term given to fluids used during tissue processing as an inter-
mediary between alcohol and paraffin wax and of course miscible
with each. Originally fluids of high refractive index such as xylene,
benzene, and toluene were employed, the tissues being rendered
transparent, hence the term 'clearing agent'. A much wider range of
media is now used, and the pedants have suggested such barbarisms
as 'de-alcoholization agents'. The term 'antemedia' has been
proposed, and this at least has something to commend it since
many of these reagents do not in fact 'clear' the tissue, but all of
them precede infiltration. Among the most popular, apart from the
trio mentioned above, are chloroform, cedarwood and other
essential oils, and carbon disulphide. The term 'clearing' is also
applied to the penultimate stage of staining, after dehydration and
prior to mounting, xylene being the most widely used reagent for
this purpose.

Clove oil

A colourless to pale yellow volatile oil which becomes darker
and thicker with age. It is sometimes used as a clearing agent.

Cobalt

Compounds of this element, e.g. the nitrate and chloride, are
sometimes used in cytological fixatives, notably for the demonstration of Golgi apparatus. Salts of cobalt are used also in methods for
the demonstration of alkaline phosphatase, aldolase, and calcium.

Cochineal

A natural dye of long standing obtained by drying and pulverizing the females of a species of tropical insect, *Coccus cacti coccinellifera*. The crude product thus extracted is sometimes used but more commonly carmine (q.v.), which is derived from cochineal treated with alum, is preferred.

Co-enzymes

A group of organic substances associated with certain enzymes, especially the dehydrogenases, as prosthetic groups attached to the essentially protein enzyme. They are sometimes referred to in this connection as diaphorases, and contain nucleic acid derivatives known as nucleotides, being closely allied to the B vitamins. They act as hydrogen carriers from substrate to acceptor, and thus perform an important catalytic function in the complex oxidation-reduction processes of tissue respiration. Two co-enzymes of histochemical importance are recognized: co-enzyme I (nicotinamide adenine dinucleotide – NAD) and co-enzyme II (nicotinamide adenine dinucleotide phosphate – NADP). Their demonstration, e.g. by monotetrazolium salts (MTT), is dependent on the transfer of hydrogen during the oxidation-reduction process to the tetrazolium salt, resulting, after chelation with cobalt chloride, in the deposition of black formazan deposits at the sites of activity.

Collagen

The ground substance of such connective tissues as bone, cartilage, and white fibrous tissue, believed to be the product of fibroblasts. Collagen fibres are very tough with great tensile strength, such tissues as tendon being largely composed of them. Its name derives from *colla* (Gk), glue, and on hydrolysis it forms gelatin from which most glues are made. It is readily digested by pepsin, but not by trypsin (*see* Elastic tissue) and swells markedly on acid treatment. Collagen fibres do not branch but tend to collect to form bundles. Histologically collagen is stained red by Van Gieson's acid fuchsin-picric acid counterstain and green (or blue) in the Masson-Mallory trichrome procedures. It is moreover birefringent in polarized light.

Colloid

A state of matter intermediate between true solutions on the one hand and suspensions on the other. Colloidal solutions may assume one of two alternative forms: the hydrosol in which the solid particles (the dispersed phase) exist in a liquid medium (the continuous phase); and the hydrogel in which the liquid droplets (the dispersed phase) are enclosed in a solid or semi-solid medium (the continuous phase). The dispersed particles, whether liquid or solid, in colloidal solution range between 1 and 100 nanometres (nm) in diameter. Suspensions are distinguished from colloids in that the dispersed solid particles in a liquid continuous phase possess a diameter greater than 100 mμ. Emulsoid sols (emulsions) are a special form of colloid, the term being confined to the combination of two immiscible fluids, such as oil and water.

The term colloid also refers to the substance found in the thyroid vesicles and manufactured by the cubical epithelial cells, its chief constituent being thyroglobulin.

Colophonium

A resin from various species of pine, sometimes dissolved in turpentine and used as a mountant instead of Canada balsam. It has also been used mixed with paraffin wax as a ringing medium, and in alcoholic solution as a differentiator of stains of the Roman-ovsky type.

Colour index

In stain chemistry and in histology, a system of numbering biological and industrial stains was introduced in 1923 and revised in 1956, in an attempt to minimize the confusion that existed regarding their nomenclature. Most common dyes have one or more synonyms, e.g., anilin blue, marine blue, soluble blue, china blue, cotton blue, water blue, and even Wasserblau, are one and the same dye. Three of these names, ostensibly for the same product, CI 707 (1st ed.) or 42755 (2nd ed.), are listed in one well-known catalogue — at different prices; the shrewd purchaser may therefore save himself a considerable amount by careful perusal of the catalogues.

Congo red

An acid disazo dye, widely used for the demonstration of amyloid, for instance, in Bennhold's and Freudenthal's methods respectively. The results tend to be somewhat nonspecific as elastic tissue also stains.

Congo red

Solubility at 20°C is 4.0 per cent in water and 1.2 per cent in alcohol.

Copper sulphate

Anhydrous cupric sulphate ($CuSO_4$) is a white or bluish-white powder employed routinely during processing of tissues at the terminal alcohol stage to ensure complete removal of the last vestiges of water; the third alcohol bath contains a layer (about ½-inch deep) of copper sulphate covered with filter paper to avoid contamination or colouration of the tissues. It also acts as an indicator of the presence of water, which will promptly convert the white anhydrous to the blue hydrated compound. In fluorescence microscopy a 5–10 per cent solution may be used as a filter for absorbing residual red light.

Corticosteroids

See Ketosteroids.

Creosote

A distillate of beechwood, colourless or light brownish, with a pungent smoky odour. It is miscible with alcohol, chloroform, ether, xylene, and various oils, but only sparingly so with water. It is used as an ingredient of Gothard's differentiator after toluidine blue or thionin in the demonstration of Nissl substance; and either alone or in conjunction with phenol and xylene for clearing celloidin or frozen sections.

Cresyl violet

A basic quinone-imine dye of the oxazin sub-group referred to often as cresyl echt violet or cresyl fast violet. It has metachromatic properties and also finds wide application in the field of nervous tissue staining, notably of Nissl substance. Cytologically it is recommended for the demonstration of sex chromatin.

Cresyl violet

Solubility at $20°C$ is 0.4 per cent in water and 0.25 per cent in alcohol.

Cross striations

Alternate light and dark bands which appear to traverse the cytoplasm of voluntary and cardiac muscle cells, when cut longitudinally. Their clarity is by no means constant from cell to cell, variations depending upon the degree of contraction and plane of section of the muscle. High-power examination by ordinary illumination, by polarized light, or by electron microscopy reveals the presence of a more detailed structure consisting of alternating bands or discs. Seen by ordinary illumination they are as follows: Dark A bands (anisotropic), with a central narrow pale core, the H (Heller) band. The A bands are separated from each other by a light isotropic I band, which itself contains a thin dark core, the Z (Zwischenscheibe) band.

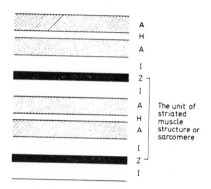

The unit of striated muscle structure or sarcomere

For recommended staining methods, *see* Muscle.

Cryostat

An apparatus for controlling temperatures at low levels; in histology, such a machine incorporates a microtome, usually of the rocking or rotary variety; it is becoming increasingly popular as a mode of obtaining frozen sections, tending to supplant the orthodox freezing microtome. It is ideally suited to small pieces of unfixed tissue, and is equipped with an anti-roll device which, coupled with the coldnesss of the microtome knife, enables flat sections to be cut and transferred easily to a clean slide, and immediately fixed and stained. The entire operation, from receipt of fresh specimen to completion of staining, may well be performed within 7 or 8 minutes; this is an appreciable saving of time compared with the classical freezing microtome methods, and hence is invaluable where rapid diagnosis is required. The apparatus also finds considerable use in work on enzyme histochemistry and in fluorescent antibody techniques, for which it was originally designed.

Crystal violet (hexamethyl pararosanilin)

A valuable basic dye of the phenyl methane family. Its uses in histology include the demonstration of Gram-positive micro-organisms and fibrin (Gram method and its modifications), neuroglial fibres (Holzer's method), and amyloid which is stained metachromatically.

Crystal violet

Solubility at 20°C is 1.43 per cent in water and 5.0 per cent in alcohol.

Cytochrome oxidase

An oxidative enzyme present in mitochondria, it acts as a catalyst in the oxidation reaction between α-naphthol and dimethyl-p-phenylenediamine to form indophenol blue (Nadi reaction). In 1958, the dimethyl-p-phenylenediamine was replaced by 4-amino-N,N-dimethylnaphthylamine (ADN) to form indonaphthol purple, a much more stable end-product, giving more precise localization. It is essential for the demonstration of this enzyme that fresh unfixed frozen sections should be used. The reactions are completely inhibited by potassium cyanide.

Cytology

That branch of histology which deals specifically with the examination and study of individual cells and their inclusions, the term generally being applied nowadays to exfoliative cytology (q.v.).

D

Dahlia

A dye, or more often an indefinite mixture of dyes, of the phenyl methane group, intermediate chemically between basic fuchsin and methyl violet. It sometimes finds application as a stain for amyloid, but seems to have little to commend it in preference to the more determinate entity, methyl violet.

Dammar

A yellowish, translucent, resinous exudate obtained from an Indonesian tree. In purified form it is used, dissolved in xylene or chloroform, as a mountant or preservative for microscopic preparations. Its refractive index is 1.520.

Dark ground microscopy

A specialized form of microscopic examination, dependent on the illumination of small transparent or unstained objects by oblique light, thus rendering them self-luminous against a dark ground. The result is achieved by the use of a special condenser, the central rays of light being obliterated and the peripheral rays passing through the object, but not entering the objective. The method of examination is of limited use in histopathology, and is restricted mainly to the diagnosis of spirochaetal infections.

De-alcoholization

See Clearing agents.

Decalcification

The removal from tissues of calcium salts, usually in the form of phosphates or carbonates in order to facilitate sectioning. Various methods may be employed, which may be summarized as follows.

(1)   Simple solution of the calcium salts in dilute mineral or organic acids, e.g., nitric, hydrochloric, formic, trichloracetic.

(2)   Electrophoresis, a modification of the above method, whereby removal of calcium is expedited by the use of an electric current; the freed calcium ions migrate to the negative electrode and the tissue remains surrounded by a virtually calcium-free acid. The heat and effervescence engendered by the reaction are thought to be factors contributory to rapid decalcification.

(3)   Ion-exchange resins, a more recently devised modification of the simple solution process, relying on the use of a polystyrene resin in conjunction with an organic acid, the resin having the power to adsorb the calcium ions so liberated.

(4)   Chelation, binding of calcium by certain organic compounds, notably ethylene diamine tetra-acetic acid (versene or sequestrene). Stress should be laid on the danger of over-decalcification, resulting in maceration of the tissues and impairment of nuclear staining. The process may be controlled either chemically with sodium or ammonium oxalate or radiographically.

Dehydration

The removal of water from tissues or from sections, the most popular agents being alcohol or, less often, acetone. Dehydration is a necessary step during processing of tissues in embedding media which are intolerant of water, such as paraffin, celloidin, and certain others. During paraffin processing it forms an essential link between aqueous media and the clearing agent which precedes wax impregnation; whereas in the celloidin technique it is used prior to alcohol-ether, which is the solvent employed for celloidin. It is normal

41

practice, in order to minimize distortion of the tissues, to use graded alcohols (e.g., 50 per cent, 70 per cent, 90 per cent) and two or three changes of absolute ethyl alcohol, the last of these containing a layer of anhydrous copper sulphate to remove any last trace of water.

The term 'dehydration' is also used in staining methods to denote removal of water from tissue sections prior to mounting. Again alcohol is normally employed, the wet section being drained or blotted, subjected to several changes of absolute ethyl alcohol, transferred to a clearing agent, usually xylene, and mounted.

Dehydrogenases

A group of oxidative enzymes present in all tissues and capable of activating an oxidation-reduction process by the removal of hydrogen from the appropriate substrate to an acceptor, usually a co-enzyme (q.v.). Several of the dehydrogenases may be demonstrated histochemically (notably by the tetrazolium salts which are capable of accepting the hydrogen so liberated), with the production of coloured formazan deposits at the sites of enzyme activity.

Dendrites

Branched protoplasmic processes of a nerve-cell or neurone which conduct impulses towards the cell, in contradistinction to the axon which conducts impulses away from the cells. Their demonstration may be effected by those methods applicable to axons.

Depigmentation

The bleaching or decolourization of a pigment, sometimes advisable in order to clarify cellular structure. For example, in a melanoma the melanin is removed either by oxidation in hydrogen peroxide or potassium permanganate, or by using nascent chlorine, liberated by the interaction of potassium chlorate and hydrochloric acid (Mayer's bleach). Haemozoin, the haematogenous pigment of malaria, may be removed by those methods used to eliminate formalin pigment, to which it is closely allied. Saturated alcoholic picric acid is probably the most effective means.

Derived lipids

A group of fatty substances, including fatty acids and cholesterol, derived by hydrolysis from neutral fats (triglycerides) and cholesterol esters respectively. Methods for the demonstration of fatty acids and cholesterol may be found under these headings.

Desoxyribonucleic acid (DNA)

One of the two complex nucleoproteins, variously known as

deoxyribonucleic acid, thymonucleic acid, or DNA — the other being ribonucleic acid or RNA (q.v.).

Nuclear chromatin is dependent for its strongly basic affinities on the presence of DNA, which on hydrolysis yields pentose sugars, phosphoric acid and the four nitrogenous bases, adenine, guanine, cytosine and thymine. It may be demonstrated specifically by the methyl green component of the Unna-Pappenheim stain, by the Feulgen reaction, by the naphthoic acid-hydrazide (NAH) method, or by fluorescence microscopy using such dyes as acridine orange.

Diamond knives

These are used in ultra-microtomy as an expensive, but in some respects advantageous, alternative to glass knives. Carefully ground and polished industrial diamonds, mounted in a block of metal, are especially preferable in dealing with hard materials such as plant tissues, bone and collagen. Once in position, the adjustment of tilt and clearance being critical, such a knife may remain set up for a long time.

Diaphorases

See Co-enzymes.

Diastase

One of several enzymes capable of digesting glycogen (q.v.). It is normally present in human saliva or may be obtained commercially as malt diastase.

Diazonium salts

A group of histochemical reagents closely related to the true dyes in that they possess the chromophoric azo $-N = N-$ group, and are capable of producing coloured derivatives by the interaction with certain enzymes or other tissue constituents, e.g., serotonin.

Diazo reaction

Certain chemical compounds, derived from the aromatic amines and closely related to the dyestuffs, have recently attained considerable importance in the realm of histochemistry. They are the di- and tetrazoniums, themselves unstable, but capable of stabilization to form double salts. In combination with phenol, indole, or imidazole groups, they are also able to produce coloured products. Such a substance is Fast Red Salt B, a diazotate of 5-nitro-anisidine, popularized by Lison and Gomori for the demonstration of argentaffin granules by virtue of their unsubstituted phenolic content; the diazonium salt is reduced to form a diazo dye. Among other diazotates sometimes used are those of o-anisidine, α-naphthylamine and o-aminoazotoluene.

Dichroism

An optical phenomenon whereby certain substances, when viewed by plane polarized light exhibit birefringency in a colour differing from the original. For example, amyloid stained by Congo red is seen, on rotation of the Nicol prisms, to be brightly birefringent, the colour changing quite suddenly at one stage of rotation from yellowish-red to a clear bright green. This characteristic colour change is peculiar to amyloid and is of considerable value in its differentiation from other Congo red-positive substances.

Differentiation

The removal of excess stain from tissue sections in order to clarify specific cell or tissue components. The sequence of procedures which entails over-staining followed by differentiation is known as 'regressive staining' (q.v.) and has largely superseded 'progressive staining', in which the degree of colouration is controlled by periodic examination. Differentiation may be carried out by dissolving excess stain or dye-lake, or by a replacement mechanism using a counterstain. Examples of the former method are weak alkalis, e.g., tap water (eosin, acid fuchsin, and other acid dyes), weak acids, e.g., 1 per cent hydrochloric (some haematoxylins, basic fuchsin, and so on), and oxidants, e.g., potassium permanganate, ferric chloride (some haematoxylins). The replacement method of differentiation is typified by the Champy-Kull technique for mitochondria (aniline acid fuchsin—toluidine blue—aurantia sequence) and by some trichrome methods.

Digitonin ($C_{56}H_{92}O_{29}$)

An organic compound derived from the same source as digitalis, employed in Windaus's method for the demonstration of free cholesterol with which it forms an insoluble complex. This reaction is dependent on the presence of a 3-β-hydroxyl group in cholesterol and similar steroids, which is absent from cholesterol esters.

Dioxan (1, 4-diethylene dioxide – $(C_2H_4)_2O_2$)

A colourless inflammable liquid with a highly poisonous vapour. It is miscible with water, alcohol, most clearing agents and paraffin wax; it may be employed therefore as a combined dehydrating and clearing agent. It causes less shrinkage than alcohol, but in mixtures with wax is extremely intolerant of traces of water.

Direct staining

A term used to denote the colouration of tissues by application of a simple solution of a dye substance without recourse to a mordant (q.v.). Common examples of such direct stains are methylene blue and neutral red (basic dyes), and eosin and acid fuchsin (acid dyes).

Disazo

See Azo dyes.

Dissociation

A method of tissue examination whereby the specimen, usually in saline or glycerine, is teased out with a dissecting needle and examined microscopically, either with reduced illumination or, better, by phase-contrast microscopy. The study of living tissues is thus possible and cellular details and movement, such as mito-chondria and mitoses, are often visible.

Dopa-oxidase

See Tyrosinase.

Double embedding

A process whereby celloidin-impregnated material is embedded in paraffin wax; serial sectioning is greatly facilitated by this means. The method is especially suited to tough or horny material, e.g., keratinized skin and chitinous substances. After fixation, tissues are dehydrated, impregnated with celloidin or a methyl benzoate-celloidin mixture, cleared in chloroform and embedded in paraffin wax.

Double refraction (*Synonyms:* Birefringence; Anisotropicity)

DPX mountant

A clear colourless synthetic mountant composed of a polystyrene (distrene), a plasticizer (tricresyl phosphate) and the solvent xylene. Its refractive index is identical with that of Canada balsam (1.524). It dries much more rapidly than Canada balsam and preserves the colour of most stained preparations well. Excess mountant may readily be peeled off when dry, but there is a danger of retraction and bubble formation, especially on thicker (celloidin) sections. A variant of this mountant, BPS, is sometimes used, the plasticizer in this case being dibutyl phthalate.

E

Ehrlich, Paul (1854–1915)

A German scientist whose work covered an immense field, primarily in immunology and chemistry, but whose main claim to fame in the histology laboratory lies in his alum haematoxylin, still after 60 years the most widely used nuclear stain.

Elastic tissue

A type of connective tissue with widespread distribution, whose fibres, as the name implies, yield easily to stretching, and regain their natural length on removal of tension. They differ from collagen fibres (q.v.) in that they are highly resistant to boiling water and alkaline solutions, but are digested by trypsin. Moreover, in bulk, elastic tissue is yellowish, whereas collagen appears glistening white. Elastic tissue is found most abundantly in arterial walls, lungs, trachea and in the dermis. Its elective demonstration may be achieved by orcein or resorcin-fuchsin and its variants, and it may also be stained with Gomori's aldehyde-fuchsin or with Verhoeff's iodine haematoxylin.

Electron microscope

An instrument similar in purpose to the light microscope but with a much higher power of resolution: the limit of resolution with a light microscope is of the order of about 2,000 Å − 1 micrometre (μm) = 10,000 Ångström units (Å); with the electron microscope details down to less than 50 Å may be observed. The principle depends on the use of a parallel beam of electrons passing through the object, which must consist of a very thin film of material (sections of less than 0.05 μm are used). On passing through the object the electrons are scattered to form an image which is then conveyed in the beam and brought to a sharp focus by a magnetic or electrostatic field, analogous to the lens system of the ordinary microscope. This greatly magnified image is then received on a fluorescent screen or photographic plate.

Electrophoresis

A term used in histological procedure to denote the utilization of an electric current in a decalcifying fluid, whereby the removal from tissues of calcium salts is accelerated, probably in large measure as a result of the heat evolved.

See Decalcification.

Embedding

The terminal stages of tissue processing, comprising the impregnation of the specimens with some fluid medium which, either by cooling or by evaporation, assumes a solid form. Common examples of the former process are paraffin and ester waxes, the tissue being subjected (after fixation, dehydration, and clearing) to several changes of the medium, after which it is 'cast', 'embedded', or 'blocked out' in a container of fresh molten wax. On cooling, this produces a block containing the tissue, which is infiltrated and surrounded by solid wax, and is thus suitable for microtomy. Essentially similar in principle are celloidin, low-viscosity nitrocellulose, and certain resins, the medium in each of these cases being employed in solutions of increasing strengths. The specimen is ultimately 'cast' in a concentrated semi-solid solution which is allowed to evaporate to hardness. Occasionally water-soluble media (e.g. gelatin and carbo-waxes) are used thus eliminating dehydration and clearing from these techniques.

Endocrine

Secreting directly into the blood stream or the lymphatic system. The term relates particularly to the ductless glands, such as the adrenals, pituitary, thyroid, pancreatic islets and the gonads (testes and ovaries).

See Exocrine.

Endogenous pigments

A group of self-coloured substances (usually yellow to dark brown) manufactured within the body; they comprise the haematogenous pigments derived from blood and the so-called autogenous pigments (melanin and the lipofuscins).

See Exogenous pigments.

Endothelium

A term given to single layers of squamous cells which line those body cavities that do not communicate with the exterior, such as the blood and lymphatic vessels, the pleural sacs and the peritoneum.

Enterochromaffin

A name given to certain cells in the stomach and more commonly in the intestines; alternatively known as argentaffin (q.v.) or Kultschitsky cells.

Enzyme

One of a number of complex organic substances, constituents of the living cell, which will catalyse a biochemical reaction in a highly specific fashion. Their *in situ* demonstration is dependent on their action on specific substrates, often in conjunction with other substances, resulting in the formation of an insoluble deposit which may be rendered visible at the site of enzyme activity. Special precautions are essential for the preservation of enzymes and the manifestation of their activity, in view of their extreme instability and rapid disappearance after cell death. Even with scrupulous care, the accurate localization of enzyme activity is considerably complicated by treatment with several reagents in sequence, each of which may bring about diffusion of the reaction products. Enzymes may be subdivided into several groups, each of them lending itself to some specialized form of treatment: (1) phosphomono-esterases, including acid and alkaline phosphatase; (2) aliesterases and cholinesterases, the former including lipases and non-specific esterases; (3) other hydrolytic enzymes, including glycosidases; and (4) oxidative enzymes, including peroxidases and dehydrogenases.

Eosin

A group of dyes, derived from fluorescein which, with the erythrosins, phloxines and rose bengals, constitute an important subdivision of the xanthene dyes. They are all acid to differing degrees and their composition, behaviour, and colour are controlled by the presence of various halogen atoms. Probably the most widely-used stain in this family is eosin Y (yellowish) which is tetrabromo fluorescein.

Eosin Y (tetrabromo fluorescein)

This stain is usually employed in aqueous solution, often as a counterstain to basic dyes such as haematoxylin; but when an alcoholic eosin is preferred, the eosin of choice is the ethyl ester. Eosin B (bluish) is occasionally used, this being a dinitro dibromo fluorescein. Apart from its intrinsic value as a plasma stain, it is one of the two vital constituents (the other being methylene blue) of the Romanovsky group with its wide haematological applications.

Solubility of eosin Y at 20°C is 41.0 per cent in water and 5.0 per cent in alcohol.

Eosinophil

Any histological structure readily stained by eosin, in particular eosinophil leucocytes. These cells may be demonstrated in tissue sections either by a weak (1/1000) eosin or, better, by chromotrope 2R.

Epinephrin (*Synonym:* Adrenalin)

Epithelium

The covering layers of the skin and mucous membranes, classified according to the shape and function of their component cells. These may be squamous, cubical, or columnar and occur sometimes

48

as a single layer of cells (simple epithelia) and sometimes as a layer several cells deep (compound epithelia). They rest, in each case, on a basement membrane which serves to separate it from the underlying connective tissue. The functions of epithelia may be protective, secretory, excretory, or sensory, and the appearance of the cells may be modified accordingly. The mucus-secreting columnar epithelium of the intestine or of the bronchus, the ciliated epithelium of the Fallopian tube and the zymogen-secreting acinar cells of the pancreas are examples of such functional modification.

Epoxy resins

A group of transparent, yellowish thermosetting resins derived from epichlorohydrin: $H_2C \overset{O}{-\!\!-} CHCH_2Cl$ and bis-phenol-A.

Bis-phenol-A

They are tending to supersede the acrylic resins in ultramicrotomy. They have the virtue of being less prone to shrinkage but, because of their greater viscosity, require a longer period for infiltration. The process is essentially similar to that using the methacrylates. Of the epoxy resins, Araldite is the most widely used.

Erythrosin

A group of dyes, in company with the eosins, phloxines, and rose bengals, which go to make up the xanthene group. They differ chemically from the eosins in that the substituent halogen atoms are of iodine rather than bromine. It is occasionally used as an alternative to eosin.

Erythrosin

Solubility at $20°C$ is 11.0 per cent in water and 2.1 per cent in alcohol.

Ester

The product of reaction between an alcohol and an acid, with special reference in histology to those reactions between higher alcohols, for example, glycerol and cholesterol, and fatty acids, notably palmitic, stearic, and oleic. The process is analogous in

49

inorganic chemistry to the production of a salt from acid + base, but differs from it in that esterification is a reversible process (hydrolysis of an ester yields fatty acid). The neutral fats or triglycerides (esters of fatty acids), in company with cholesterol esters, constitute the subgroup of simple lipids.

Esterases
> *See* Aliesterases.

Ester wax
> An embedding medium of comparatively recent introduction (devised by Steedman in 1947), harder and more translucent than paraffin wax but with a lower mp (about 47°C). It has moreover a wider range of miscibility; ethanol, isopropanol, acetone, aniline, as well as the usual wax solvents are miscible with it. Cedarwood oil, cellosolve and dioxan have also been recommended. Its prime application is in the field of enzyme work.

Ethanolamine
> *See* Phospholipids.

Ether, ethyl (diethyl ether – $C_2H_5OC_2H_5$)
> Usually known simply as ether, it is a volatile, highly inflammable, colourless, sweet-smelling, mobile liquid. In histology it has a variety of uses: (1) as an anaesthetic for laboratory animals; (2) as a fat solvent; (3) mixed with an equal volume of ethyl alcohol as a solvent for celloidin and other nitrocelluloses; and (4) with glycerol as a differentiator for polychrome methylene blue.

Ether, petroleum
> An explosive, highly inflammable, poisonous mixture of hydrocarbons, mostly pentanes and hexanes. It figures occasionally in processing methods as an alternative to the common clearing agents, notably in enzyme techniques.

Euparal
> A mounting medium composed of a mixture of sandarac resin, eucalyptus, camphor, phenyl salicylate and paraldehyde. It has a refractive index of 1.483, lower than that of most of the resinous media, and has the advantage that sections may be mounted from alcohol (90 per cent–100 per cent) as well as from xylene. A green variant containing a copper salt is alleged to intensify the colour of haematoxylin-stained sections.

Eutectic point
> The lowest freezing point obtainable when two or more

substances, capable of reducing each other's freezing point, are mixed together to form a frozen solid.

Exfoliative cytology

A branch of histological technique which deals with the examination of cells that have been removed deliberately, or have become detached spontaneously from their original environment. The cells may be found in body fluids such as sputum, urine, pleural effusions, cystic contents etc., or they may be obtained by epithelial scrapings (buccal and vaginal smears). These methods are of especial value in the diagnosis of malignant disease, in chromosome studies, and in hormone assay.

See also Papanicolaou.

Exocrine

A term applied to those glands whose secretion is conveyed by means of ducts either into the alimentary tract or directly or indirectly to the exterior. Examples of exocrine glands are the breast, the pancreas (apart from the islets of Langerhans), the sebaceous and sweat glands of the skin, and the prostate and salivary glands.

See also Endocrine.

Exogenous pigments

A heterogeneous group of coloured substances, assimilated directly or indirectly from without the body. It includes those pigments derived from the diet (the carotenoids, precursors of vitamin A), those that arise as the result of environment or occupational hazards (e.g. carbon, silica), and the miscellaneous group of tattoo-pigments, vegetable or mineral.

See Endogenous pigments.

Eye

This organ poses difficult problems of sectioning; it demands very careful processing in view of the diverse consistency of its component parts and their tendency to separate from each other. Various embedding media have been suggested, among them polyester resins as well as paraffin and ester waxes and celloidin. Fixation may be carried out, preferably by injection and subsequent immersion in formalin, formol-sublimate, Bouin, or Zenker's fluids. The last two are of course unsuitable for museum specimens. Following fixation, which should be as short as possible, the eye should be washed, frozen, and bisected with a sharp scalpel or razor-blade, and processed and embedded in the medium selected. It is essential to use a very sharp knife to obtain good sections with minimal separation

of the constituent parts or powdering of the lens. This latter hazard
may sometimes be overcome when cutting paraffin sections by
moistening the surface of the block. Sections are liable moreover
to become detached from the slide during staining; this may be
avoided by covering with a film of thin celloidin.

F

Farrant's medium

An aqueous mountant, containing gum arabic, glycerol and
arsenous oxide, and therefore very poisonous. Its refractive index
is 1.436. The addition of potassium acetate renders it less acid and
decreases its tendency to 'bleed' methyl violet.

Fast green FCF

An acid dye of the phenyl methane group, similar in composition
and behaviour to light green SF, but as the name suggests less
prone to fading. Its main use is as a counterstain in the trichrome
group of techniques.

Fast green FCF

Solubility at 20°C is 16.0 per cent in water and 0.35 per cent in
alcohol.

Fat

A term used loosely to denote any tissue of a lipid nature, either
macroscopically to mean adipose tissue or, histologically, the
complete range of lipids — simple, compound, and derived (q.v.).
See also Neutral fats; Fatty acids; Phospholipids; Galactolipids;
Cholesterol.

Fatty acids

Those lipids which may be derived from the simple and compound
lipids by hydrolysis. They form two series: the saturated, with the
general formula $C_nH_{2n+1}COOH$, and the unsaturated, usually
$C_nH_{2n-1}COOH$. The saturated fatty acids include simple compounds such as formic acid (H.COOH) and acetic acid (CH_3COOH),

but of those occurring in mammalian tissue palmitic ($C_{15}H_{31}COOH$) and stearic ($C_{17}H_{35}COOH$) acids are of major importance histologically. The unsaturated fatty acids form a smaller and less significant group, the chief naturally-occurring one being oleic acid ($C_{17}H_{33}COOH$). Fatty acids in tissues may be demonstrated by dyes such as the Sudan group and Nile blue, by osmium tetroxide (Marchi's method for degenerate myelin), and specifically by Fischler's copper acetate-haematoxylin method. Polariscopic examination is sometimes helpful.

Ferric chloride ($FeCl_3.6H_2O$)

A brownish-yellow, deliquescent, lumpy compound used as a mordant for haematoxylin (e.g. Weigert's and Verhoeff's haematoxylins); in conjunction with potassium ferricyanide as Schmorl's reagent for reducing substances; and as the active agent in the Vulpian reaction for chromaffin tissue.

Ferric iron

See Haemosiderin.

Ferrous iron

See Haemosiderin.

Feulgen

The reaction bearing this name is regarded as a specific test for desoxyribonucleic acid (DNA), q.v. It is dependent on mild acid hydrolysis of the nucleic acids, whereby reactive aldehyde groups are released. Such a liberation probably occurs also with ribonucleic acid, but much more slowly; the duration of hydrolysis must not, therefore, be excessive. The aldehydes thus freed may be visualized by Schiff's reagent (q.v.).

Fibrin

A whitish insoluble protein derived from plasma fibrinogen, associated particularly with acute inflammatory conditions. Its histological demonstration may be effected in several ways: by the Gram-Weigert crystal violet method and subsequent differentiation in aniline-xylene; by Mallory's phosphotungstic acid haematoxylin, which gives a powerful but non-specific demonstration; and by Lendrum's picro-Mallory methods, which probably give the most satisfactory and unequivocal pictures. Fibrin undergoes digestion with trypsin even after formalin fixation, and may thus be differentiated from fibrinoid and collagen.

Fibrinoid

An indeterminate group of substances resembling fibrin and

found in arteriosclerotic vessels, placenta, etc. It is probably formed by the precipitation of an acid mucopolysaccharide with a basic protein and possesses similar staining reactions, for the most part, to those of fibrin. A probable exception is the Gomori reticulin technique, by which fibrinoid is demonstrated positively and fibrin itself excluded. Moreover fibrinoid, in contrast to fibrin, is not digestible with trypsin.

Fixation

The process whereby tissues are preserved and rendered resistant to the action of reagents to which they may be subjected later. The primary aim of fixation is the rapid killing or fixing of the cells, so that a reasonable approximation to their appearance during life is achieved. It follows from this that any degenerative changes, autolytic and putrefactive, which inevitably commence on removal of tissue from the parent organism, must be arrested with minimal delay, and the tissue placed immediately in the selected fixative solution. Such selection is governed by the nature of the examination required, whether it be from the standpoint of general architecture or of individual cell structure. An adequate volume of fixative (at least 20 times that of the tissue) should always be used. The physical action and properties of fixing agents will be found under the appropriate headings.

Fluorescein

A yellow acid dye of the xanthene group, noteworthy as being the parent substance of the eosins, erythrosins, and allied dyes. Its staining power is very limited, but its fluorescent properties are extremely powerful, even in very weak dilutions, but more especially in ultra-violet light.

Fluorescein

Solubility at $20°C$ is 0.03 per cent in water and 2.21 per cent in alcohol.

Fluorescence microscopy

Fluorescence is the property whereby certain substances may be excited by light rays of one wave length and emit light of a different and longer wave length. This differs from phosphorescence in that the phenomenon ceases when the light stimulus is cut off. Usually the excitant light is in the ultra-violet range (below 400 nm), the induced fluorescent light falling within the visible spectrum.

Fluorescence exists in two forms: primary (auto-) fluorescence, an inherent property of certain substances; and secondary fluorescence, induced by the application of fluorochrome dyes. Examples of the former are Vitamin A and elastic fibres, and of the latter DNA and RNA (acridine orange), acid-fast bacilli (auramine), and amyloid (thioflavine T). The equipment, which may be relatively simple, consists essentially of a microscope, ultra-violet or blue light source, and a two filter-system; the latter consists of an exciter filter between light source and object (to eliminate all light above 400 nm and permit the passage exclusively of ultra-violet light), and a barrier filter, situated in the eyepiece (to absorb ultra-violet light and so avoid the danger of retinal damage).

Formaldehyde (HCHO)

A colourless gas with a pungent odour, soluble in water to about 55 per cent, and prepared by the oxidation of methyl alcohol over heated metal. It is a powerful reducing agent, especially in the presence of alkali, and oxidizes slowly to form formic acid. It is a potent antiseptic and disinfectant, and an excellent preservative. This last property makes it the most widely used histological fixative. It is available commercially in aqueous solution (about 40 per cent), which is known as 'formalin'; this is normally diluted with about ten parts of water. The tissue proteins are not precipitated by formalin, as is the case with most fixing agents, but form addition compounds with it. It is popular for several reasons: it is cheap; it renders tissues firm but not brittle, thus permitting easy sectioning; it allows the natural colour of specimens to be restored for museum mounting, provided fixation time is not unduly prolonged. For general microtomy the length of fixation is not highly critical, excellent staining and impregnation pictures often being obtained after several months; it may be followed by a very wide range of staining methods; and although it is often used alone, it is also included in many fixing mixtures. The main disadvantages of formalin are: (1) it is intensely irritating to the mucous membranes, and exposure may also give rise to a persistent dermatitis; and (2) it becomes acid on standing, owing to the formation of formic acid, and this has a deleterious effect on nuclear staining and also promotes the formation of acid formaldehyde haematin ('formalin pigment', q.v.). This tendency may be counteracted and the pH stabilized in the diluted fixing solution by the addition of a soluble buffer.

Formalin

The name given to a concentrated aqueous solution (about 37 per cent by weight or 40 g/100 ml of solution) of formaldehyde gas. This is usually known as commercial formalin. The terms formalin and formaldehyde may give rise to a certain amount of confusion, and reference to percentage solutions should perhaps be designated in terms of formaldehyde. Thus for example the term '10 per cent formalin' might well be abandoned in favour of '4 per cent formaldehyde'.

See also Formaldehyde and Acid formaldehyde haematin.

Formalin pigment

See Acid formaldehyde haematin.

Formic acid (H.COOH)

A naturally-occurring fatty acid, first observed in 1670 as a product arising from the distillation of ants (L. *formica*); it is also the active principle of some stinging plants (e.g., Nettle). It is a colourless liquid with a pungent smell and powerful caustic properties, and is a strong reducing agent. Its main histological application is found in decalcification methods, where it may be used in straight aqueous solution (usually 5 per cent) or in conjunction with formalin (5 per cent formic acid in 4 per cent saline formaldehyde, known as Gooding and Stewart's fluid).

Freeze drying

A method of tissue preservation alternative to orthodox fixation and dehydration, whereby small portions of tissue are rapidly frozen or 'quenched' in isopentane, and cooled by immersion in liquid nitrogen to about $-170°C$. The tissue is then quickly transferred to a vacuum chamber and the ice removed by sublimation to a vapour trap, this procedure being carried out at a temperature of about $-35°C$. The distance between the tissue and the condensing surface of the vapour trap largely controls the speed and effectiveness of desiccation, but this is usually complete within 48 hours. When fully dried the tissue may be directly impregnated, still in vacuo, in paraffin or water-soluble wax. Sections should be cut slightly thicker than usual and either mounted from warm mercury or attached direct to warm albuminized slides by finger pressure. Water mounting is contra-indicated because of disintegration of the unfixed tissue, but should fixation be desirable, sections may be floated on to warm formol-saline. Freeze drying techniques lend themselves especially to the demonstration of enzymes and of mitochondria.

Freeze substitution

A group of techniques that may be used as an inexpensive alternative to freeze drying (q.v.). In essence the methods entail rapid quenching, for example in isopentane at $-160°C$, after which the tissues are transferred to a dehydrating fixative at $-70°C$. Suggested fixatives are 1 per cent mercuric chloride or 1 per cent picric acid in ethyl alcohol, or 1 per cent osmium tetroxide in acetone for one week. Following this the fixed tissues are transferred either to alcohol at room temperature (in the case of alcoholic fixatives), or to acetone at $-70°C$ (in the case of the osmic-acetone fixation). They are then cleared, embedded in paraffin or ester wax, sectioned, and stained accordingly. Freeze-substitution methods are superior, at least theoretically, to the standard methods of fixation, in that the initial quenching immediately arrests cellular activity and autolytic and putrefactive changes. Moreover, immersion in the cold fixative over a period of gradual thaw ensures that penetration and fixation occur contemporaneously.

Frozen sections

For the majority of histological purposes, embedding media such as paraffin wax, celloidin and resins are used in order to provide support for the tissues during section cutting. Such techniques however usually entail the use of heat or of reagents which may dissolve certain tissue constituents (for example, lipids). Moreover, some measure of shrinkage and distortion is unavoidable. These disadvantages may be largely overcome by the use of frozen sections which may be obtained by congelation of the tissue by compressed carbon dioxide, sections being cut on a freezing microtome. Alternatively, the cold microtome or cryostat (q.v.) or the thermomodule (q.v.) may be used. The main applications of frozen sections are as follows: (1) for the demonstration of lipids and of enzymes; (2) for the rapid diagnosis of biopsy and other urgent material, stained preparations being available in 10 minutes or less; (3) for the examination of material from the nervous system, especially in association with the metallic impregnation methods.

See also Microtomy.

Fuchsin acid

See Acid fuchsin.

Fuchsin basic

See Basic fuchsin.

Fungi

The examination of fungi in tissues is sometimes required, and the method of choice is governed largely by the nature of the fungus. Commonly used are periodic acid-Schiff modifications such as Bauer and Gridley, Heidenhain's iron haematoxylin, the metachromatic and other mucin stains, the Gram techniques and some silver impregnations.

G

Galactolipids

Known alternatively as glycolipids or cerebrosides, they constitute a subgroup of the compound lipids. On hydrolysis they yield a carbohydrate (usually galactose), a fatty acid, and the nitrogenous base sphingosine. These lipids are usually coexistent with the phospholipids (q.v.) and are especially abundant in nervous tissue. Three cerebrosides at least are known: phrenosin, kerasin and nervon, which differ only in the nature of the fatty acid yielded on hydrolysis. Their demonstration is not easily effected, but a positive reaction is given with the PAS and PFAS methods (q.v.) as well as with the Sudan stains. The phospholipids may also be stained by these methods, but differentiation between the two groups can be achieved by solubility tests, hot acetone readily dissolving the galactolipids and leaving the phospholipids untouched.

Gallocyanin

One of the oxazin subgroup of quinone-imine dyes; in company with celestine blue, which it closely resembles, it is a useful nuclear stain and, like celestine blue, the staining solution relies on laking of the dye with iron or chrome alum. Perhaps its main application is in the demonstration of Nissl substance which is stained very effectively by it.

Gallocyanin

Gamete

A term applied to the reproductive cell, in the female to the ovum, in the male to the spermatozoon, the two uniting to form a zygote.

Gamma rays

Electromagnetic rays of very short wave-length emitted during the disintegration of radioactive substances.

Ganglion

A term applied to a collection of nerve cells serving as a centre of nervous activity, for instance, the spinal ganglia situated on the posterior roots of the spinal cord. The constituent cells have typically a rounded nucleus with a prominent nucleolus and an abundant cytoplasm containing chromidial material, intracellular fibrils, and often granules of lipofuscin pigment. Basic dyes such as haematoxylin, celestine blue, gallocyanin, and dyes of the thiazin group (thionin and toluidin blue) may be used to demonstrate the cytoplasmic chromidia. The intracellular neurofibrils and lipofuscin pigments are dealt with under their respective headings.

See also Lipofuscin; Neurofibrils.

Geiger (or Geiger-Müller) counter

An instrument for detecting ionizing radiations, such as alpha, beta and gamma rays. It consists essentially of an axial tungsten wire anode surrounded by a cylindrical conducting cathode mounted in a glass tube containing gas at low pressure. The electrical impulses that arise on the passage of ionizing particles through the tube are amplified and registered by a mechanical counter.

Gelatin

A protein obtained by boiling various animal tissues, notably bone, and existing as a firm colourless transparent substance, quite brittle when dry and swelling and softening on exposure to water. It is readily soluble in warm water in all proportions. The physical state of gelatin, whether sol or gel, is governed normally by temperature, the sol representing the warmer, the gel the cooler phase. On exposure to formaldehyde, however, this property of reversibility is destroyed, a permanent solid being produced. A strong solution of gelatin may be used as an embedding medium for fragmentary or friable tissues as a prelude to frozen section, or for the preparation of giant sections by the Gough and Wentworth method; weaker solutions may be used as section adhesives or as aqueous mountants in conjunction with glycerine. It finds application in museum mounting either for coating delicate structures or for filling hollow spaces, such as stomach or intestine. It is also used as an injection medium containing one or more soluble dyes for the demonstration of vascular systems of organs such as lung, kidney, or placenta.

Gene

One of a series of units in the chromosome, controlling the inherited characteristics of an organism. Each gene occupies a particular point in linear order on the chromosome. It is self-reproducible on division of the cell, and is regarded as being a special molecular arrangement of the nucleoproteins which go to form DNA. Genes are as a rule highly stable, but mutate on rare occasions.

Gentian violet

A mixture of dyes of the phenyl methane group, the identity and proportions of the components varying widely. It resembles methyl violet, but usually contains lower homologues of the rosanilin group and sometimes the higher homologue, crystal violet, together with variable amounts of dextrin. No useful purpose seems to be served by retaining so inconstant a mixture, and its undoubted obsolescence is to be encouraged since its functions are fully covered by crystal violet.

Giant sections

Sections of whole organs such as lung or kidney are sometimes called for. The most popular technique is that devised by Gough and Wentworth which, after fixation and prolonged washing, requires embedding in gelatin, followed by sectioning on a special large microtome at $300-400 \mu m$. The sections are then laid on perspex sheets and covered with filter paper to which they adhere. When dry, they may be stored permanently in book form.

Glia

See Neuroglia.

Glucose-6-phosphatase

A specific and highly sensitive enzyme of the phosphatase group, occurring in liver, kidney and intestines. It may be demonstrated by methods of the Gomori lead nitrate type such as that of Wachstein and Meisel, the incubation being carried out at pH 6.7. Fresh unfixed or cryostat sections should be used, as fixation in formalin destroys this enzyme. This property has been utilized in order to differentiate it from acid and alkaline phosphatases which are more resistant to the effects of formalin. Alternatively, an inhibitor such as sorbitan-6-phosphate may be used.

β-Glucuronidase

An enzyme of the glycosidase group, of widespread occurrence in mammalian tissues, particularly in liver, kidney and spleen. Its biochemical role is not yet fully understood, but it may well be concerned with steroid metabolism. Several methods for its demonstration have been devised, of which the most reliable is probably that of Hayashi, using naphthol AS-BI glucuronide on prefixed cryostat sections at a pH of about 5.2.

Glycerol (Glycerin $CH_2OH.CHOH.CH_2OH$)

A trihydroxy alcohol obtained by the hydrolysis of neutral fats. It is a clear colourless syrupy liquid with a warm sweet taste, miscible with water and alcohol, and explosive on contact with strong oxidants such as hydrogen peroxide and potassium permanganate. It has numerous uses in histology: (1) as an aqueous mountant in conjunction with gelatin; (2) as an adhesive with egg albumin; (3) as a clearing agent in museum mounting, e.g., in Dawson's method for skeletal structure, and also as a constituent of museum mountants; (4) as an ingredient of some alum haematoxylins to minimize evaporation; and (5) in paraffin embedding to prevent adhesion of the cast paraffin block to its mould.

Glycogen $(C_6H_{10}O_5)_n$

A polysaccharide occurring naturally in the animal body, constituting the carbohydrate reservoir. It is synthesized and stored in the liver and skeletal muscles, and is converted by the liver into glucose as required by the body tissues. On contraction of the muscles it is converted into lactic acid which in the presence of oxygen from the blood is mainly reconverted into glycogen. Glycogen is extremely labile, being converted into glucose very rapidly after death. Fixation should therefore be prompt; a fixative containing picric acid (Bouin) or, alternatively, formol saline may be used. For histochemical assessment the freeze-drying technique is preferable. Its histological demonstration may be effected in several ways: (1) by the classical Best's carmine method which, although empirical, gives a highly specific and colourful result; (2) by the Schiff group, using oxidants such as periodic acid, chromic acid, or lead tetra-acetate (all of these methods being positive not only for glycogen but for a wide range of other substances); (3) by silver impregnation, e.g., by Gomori's methenamine silver, to which similar criticisms apply; and (4) by iodine methods, which again lack specificity and are perhaps less attractive from aesthetic and photographic points of view. Stress should be laid on the necessity in all of these methods for control sections; a known positive section e.g., of carrot-fed rabbit liver) in order to check the efficacy of the reagents; and a parallel series of diastase-treated sections for comparison with the untreated test sections.

61

Glycosidases

The only member of this enzyme group with appreciable histo-chemical significance is β-glucuronidase (q.v.).

Goblet cells

Columnar epithelial cells which derive their name from their ovoid shape when charged with mucin. They occur throughout the columnar epithelium of the alimentary tract, especially in the ileum and the rectum. They are also found in the pseudo-stratified columnar epithelium of the bronchus. They may be well demonstrated by the methods for mucin (q.v.).

Gold chloride

A good deal of confusion exists regarding the nature of compounds of gold with chlorine. Brown gold chloride is in fact the acid trichloride, $AuCl_3HCl.4H_2O$, and is referred to sometimes as chloro-auric acid. Yellow gold chloride, according to the authoritative Merck Index, has indeed no separate identity, but is a mixture of the above brown variety with sodium chloride; it is accordingly referred to as gold sodium chloride. The percentage of gold in the brown variety is about 50 per cent; in the yellow, usually about 30 per cent. Gold chloride forms the basis for certain metallic impregnation methods, of which the best known is Cajal's gold chloride-sublimate for astrocytes. For this purpose the stronger brown salt is to be advocated. The yellow salt is the one normally cited for 'toning' sections impregnated with silver compounds, but the brown salt is equally satisfactory for this purpose.

Golgi apparatus

A delicate intracytoplasmic fibrillary network which takes its name from Camillo Golgi, an eminent Italian histologist (1844–1926). Evidence regarding both its chemical composition and its function tends to be circumstantial, but it is generally accepted as being at least partially lipid and concerned with the mechanism of secretion. Numerous methods for its demonstration have been devised, both by Golgi and by subsequent workers. They fall into three main categories, employing respectively osmium tetroxide, silver nitrate and Sudan black.

Gram, Hans Christian Joachim (1853–1938)

A Danish physician who introduced the classical staining method for the differential demonstration of micro-organisms, which bears his name. The method has in fact become the basis for the identification and classification of most bacteria, whereby they may be subdivided into Gram-positive and Gram-negative groups. The method consists essentially of an initial methyl violet stain, with post-mordanting in iodine, followed by differentiation in one of several fluids, e.g. acetone or alcohol, and subsequent counterstaining with a contrasting, usually red, dye. Many modifications of Gram's original method have been devised, some with special application to histopathology and the demonstration of micro-organisms in tissue sections. One important variant of the method, that of Weigert, utilizing aniline-xylene as the decolourizing fluid, is widely used for staining fibrin.

Ground sections

Thin slices of undecalcified hard tissues such as bone, teeth and gallstones are sometimes called for. Modern microtomy techniques largely supersede the older methods of grinding, but the latter have the advantage of being adaptable to blocks of virtually unlimited size. Maceration of the softer material from such tissues as bone is a necessary preliminary, after which a thin slice may be cut with a fine saw. The opposing faces are then carefully ground to the required thinness and polished, using carborundum or another abrasive. Stability may be lent to the material by prior impregnation with copal varnish dissolved in chloroform and allowed to evaporate to hardness. The thin slices thus obtained may be dehydrated, dried and mounted unstained in balsam.

Guarnieri bodies

Inclusion bodies associated with vaccinia and smallpox lesions. They are demonstrable in tissue sections owing to their acidophil reaction by such methods as Lendrum's phloxine-tartrazine, Mann's methyl blue-eosin and, perhaps best, by Macchiavello's basic fuchsin-citric acid.

Gum arabic (gum acacia)

The resinous exudate of several species of African acacia, notably of Kordofan in the Sudan. It occurs in the form of spheroidal tears, is soluble in water, glycerol, and propylene glycol, but not in ethyl alcohol. It forms the basis for water mountants such as Apáthy and Farrant, and is an ingredient of Hamilton's freezing mixture (q.v.).

H

Haemalum

A term associated especially with Mayer, denoting a solution of haematoxylin combined with an alum mordant.

Haematein

The active staining principle of haematoxylin of which it is the oxidized form.

See also Haematoxylin.

Haematoidin

The bile pigments, bilirubin and biliverdin (q.v.).

Haematoxylin

Undoubtedly the most important stain at the histologist's disposal and one of the few remaining natural dyes in routine use. Crystalline haematoxylin is obtained by distillation with ether of the commercial extract of the heart-wood of a tree indigenous to Central and South America, similar to our own gorse, of the family Cesalpiniaceae. Two criteria are necessary before the powder can be utilized as a stain: (1) oxidation to haematein which occurs spontaneously, but slowly, and may be expedited chemically by such oxidants as potassium permanganate, sodium iodate, mercuric oxide, etc.; and (2) mordanting (q.v.) with either metallic salts (e.g. iron) or with alums. The generally accepted formula for haematoxylin is:

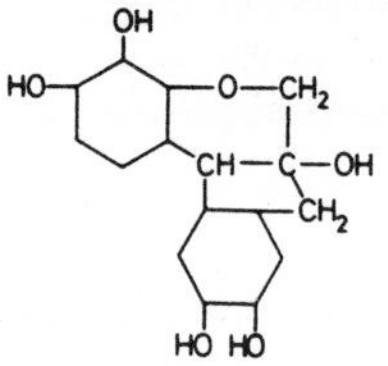

Haematoxylin

and for haematein:

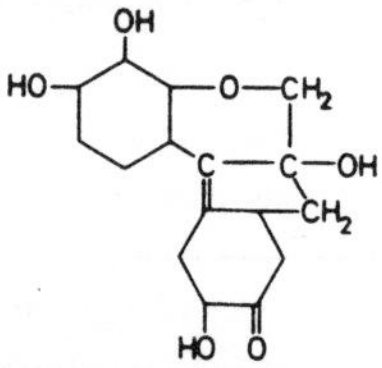

Haematein

Haematoxylin in its oxidized form (haematein), and in combination with an appropriate mordant, is a powerful basic dye, widely used as a nuclear stain with such solutions as those of Ehrlich and of Weigert and Heidenhain. In the last of these it is adaptable by varying the degree of differentiation to the demonstration of cytoplasmic constituents, e.g., mitochondria and muscle striations.

Haemofuscin

A term applied by von Recklinghausen (1899) to an iron-free pigment occurring in cases of haemochromatosis in conjunction with iron pigments. Its behaviour seems to be identical with that of the lipofuscin pigments (q.v.), and there would appear to be no valid argument for regarding it as a separate entity.

Haemoglobin

The successful histological demonstration of haemoglobin is dependent on fixation in buffered formalin, followed usually by a peroxidase technique such as the benzidine method of Lepehne-Pickworth or the leuco-patent blue of Lison-Dunn.

Haemosiderin

The name given to 'iron' pigments, a breakdown product of haemoglobin, and probably consisting of protein in combination with hydrated ferric oxide, $Fe(OH)_3$. It may be found intracellularly in haematomas, infarcts, and other conditions where haemolysis occurs, notably in haemochromatosis, and it is almost invariably present in the ferric form. It is soluble in strong acids, but this property is diminished by fixation in neutral formalin. It is visible in unstained sections as a yellow to dark-brown granular pigment, and may be demonstrated histologically by Perls' method: potassium ferrocyanide and hydrochloric acid, either together or in sequence, forming ferric ferrocyanide, $Fe_4[Fe(CN)_6]_3$, or Prussian blue. Sections mounted in Canada balsam are prone to fade, but may be revived by treatment with hydrogen peroxide. A plastic mountant is however recommended. Alternative methods of demonstration are Humphrey's dinitroso-resorcinol (giving a permanent dark-green colour), or Macallum's method using fresh aqueous haematoxylin, after liberation of the inorganic iron by treatment with dilute acid.

Haemozoin

See Malarial pigment.

Half-life

The time taken for the activity of a radioactive substance to decay to one-half of its original value; for instance, Carbon 14 (C^{14}) has a half-life of 5,600 years, Strontium 90 (Sr^{90}) 28 years and Iodine 131 (I^{131}) 8.1 days.

Hamilton's freezing mixture

A syrup used in frozen section techniques for the support of the tissue block during section-cutting, and imparting to it a firm rubbery consistency. Its use is thought by some workers to facilitate sectioning and to minimize the formation of large ice crystals. The mixture is composed of cane sugar, gum arabic and distilled water.

Hassall's corpuscles

These are bodies found exclusively in the thymus medulla,

65

comprising a rounded acidophil structure varying in diameter from 30 to 100 μm and composed of degenerate, often hyalinized, cells concentrically arranged. Calcium is sometimes present.

Heart

A roughly conical, thick muscular, rhythmically contracting organ lying within the thorax and surrounded by the pericardium. It maintains the circulation of the blood by its pumping action. It comprises four chambers, the right and left auricles and ventricles, and four valves, the mitral, tricuspid, aortic, and pulmonary. Venous blood collected from the body via the venae cavae passes into the right auricle, through the tricuspid valve into the right ventricle, thence through the pulmonary valve and artery to the lungs for oxygenation; it returns via the pulmonary veins into the left auricle and through the mitral valve into the left ventricle, and finally via the aortic valve into the aorta for distribution throughout the body. The musculature of the heart, or myocardium, is composed of striated muscle fibres with central nuclei, and therefore displays some characteristics of both voluntary and involuntary muscle.

Heiffor knife

A bi-concave microtome knife of 'cut-throat' razor type, but with a fixed, rigid handle, devised for use with rocking microtomes.

Helly, Konrad (1875–)

Swiss pathologist noted for the fixative that bears his name. It contains potassium dichromate and mercuric chloride in aqueous solution to which formalin is added immediately before use; it is commonly recommended for bone-marrow and other haemopoietic tissues, and for mitochondria.

Herapathite

Quinine iodosulphate, $4C_{20}H_{24}N_2O_2.3H_2SO_4.2HI.2I_2.6H_2O$, a pale olive-green compound in plate-like crystals, with powerful polarizing properties, utilized in science and in industry in the manufacture of polaroid material.

Hexamine $(CH_2)_6N_4$

Variously known as hexamethylene-tetramine or methenamine, it is obtained by the reaction between ammonia and formaldehyde. It is a colourless crystalline solid, soluble in water to give an alkaline solution. Histologically it is used in conjunction with silver nitrate for the demonstration of argentaffin cells, glycogen, melanin, lipofuscins, etc.

Highman's mountant

A variant of Apáthy's water-soluble mounting medium, sodium

chloride or potassium acetate being added to the original formula. Its special advantage lies in its application to methyl violet-stained amyloid preparations, wherein it prevents, or at least slows down, the customary diffusion or 'bleeding' of stain.

Histiocytes

Phagocytic cells of the connective tissues and important members of the reticulo-endothelial system, known sometimes as fixed macrophages or resting wandering cells. They are related to the von Kupffer cells of the liver, the reticulum cells of the lymphatic tissues, and the microglia of the brain, which are sometimes referred to as cerebral histiocytes. They may be seen to possess elaborate branched processes, provided that an appropriate metallic impregnation, e.g. the Weil-Davenport technique, is employed.

Histochemistry

That branch of biology that is concerned with the microscopic recognition and localization in tissues, by appropriate chemical reactions, of the various products formed or transformed by them, and the deduction therefrom of their metabolic action.

Histology (Gk *histos,* tissue + *logos,* a treatise)

That branch of biological science which deals with the minute cellular structure of both normal and pathological tissues.

Histopathology

That section of histology which is concerned with the study of diseased tissues – pathological histology.

Honing

The process whereby sharpness is restored to a blunt or damaged knife-edge. Various types of natural and artificial stone of varying degrees of abrasiveness may be used, the edge of the knife being moved back and forth across the surface of the hone until the damage has been repaired and the keenness restored. Some form of lubricant (oil, detergent, or water) is usually required. Commonly used are the Belgian, Arkansas, Aloxite and Carborundum hones. Many automatic knife-sharpening machines are now available, the majority of which utilize plate-glass wheels or discs, in conjunction with abrasive powders, for honing purposes.
See also Abrasive powder.

Hormones

Those substances secreted by ductless glands into the blood, and by this means conveyed to other organs in order to stimulate specialized activities. Their chemical nature may be protein (as in insulin and the pituitary hormones), steroid (adrenal, cortical and sex hormones), or phenolic (adrenalin).

See also Pancreas, Pituitary, Ketosteroids.

Hortega, Pío del Río (1882–1945)

A Spanish histologist and pupil of Cajal (q.v.) with whom he was associated in research into the nature and demonstration of nervous tissue components, more especially the glial elements. Impregnation with silver solutions formed the basis for most of his work, and he devised numerous techniques which have paved the way for subsequent workers in this field.

Hyaluronic acid

A complex acid mucopolysaccharide polymer of acetyl-glucosamine and glucuronic acid. It occurs in synovial fluid, vitreous humour, the ground substance of connective tissues, the umbilical cord, and in the filtrates of some bacteria; it may be demonstrated histologically by Alcian blue, PAS, and specifically by Hale's dialysed iron technique. In all such techniques it is essential that the test section should be accompanied by a parallel section that has been subjected to prior treatment with hyaluronidase, which will remove hyaluronic acid and chondroitin sulphates. Any material that is seen to be positive in the test and negative in the hyaluronidase-treated control section may reasonably be assumed to contain hyaluronic acid or a chondroitin sulphate.

Hyaluronidase

See Hyaluronic acid.

Hydrochloric acid (HCl)

A reagent with numerous uses in histology, of which the most important are: (1) as a differentiator of basic dyes, such as haematoxylin; (2) as a decalcifying agent; (3) for the hydrolysis of sections in the Feulgen reaction for DNA; (4) for the unmasking of ferric salts in the Perls' Prussian blue reaction; and (5) in high concentration for the maceration of tissues, e.g. in museum mounting techniques.

Hydrogen peroxide (H_2O_2)

A powerful oxidant available commercially in 30 per cent aqueous solution (100 volumes of oxygen) or in 3 per cent solution (10 volumes of oxygen). Concentrated hydrogen peroxide is a clear, colourless unstable fluid, decomposing violently in the presence of even small traces of impurities, with the explosive generation of large quantities of oxygen. Contact with the skin or eyes should be meticulously avoided. Its oxidant properties are utilized in histology as a ripener for some haematoxylin solutions; as a bleaching agent for certain pigments, notably melanin; for the conversion of bilirubin into biliverdin; for the demonstration of haemoglobin by the oxidation of benzidine, etc.

Hydrophilic

A term given to those 'masked' lipids, shown by chemical analysis to be present in considerable quantity in all tissues, but not demonstrable by the Sudan dyes. These lipids exist in combination with non-lipid elements of an aqueous or protein nature. They are sometimes referred to as 'heterophasic' lipids, and form the major part of the compound lipids, which are abundant in mitochondria and other cellular inclusions and, more overtly, in such substances as myelin.

See also Hydrophobic.

Hydrophobic

A term describing those 'homophasic' lipids, such as the fat droplets of storage cells, existing as separate entities, composed solely of lipid, and bounded by a hydrophobic or water-repellent surface. These lipid droplets of continuous phase are readily demonstrable by the Sudan techniques, whose principle is the greater solubility of the dye in the lipid than in the dye solvent.

See also Hydrophilic.

Hydroquinone $(C_6H_4(OH)_2)$

A photographic reducer that may be utilized for analogous purposes in histology, namely, the reduction of sections or blocks of tissue after impregnation with silver compounds. It is employed for example in the da Fano-Cajal group of methods for the block impregnation of Golgi apparatus, and in Dieterle's method for spirochaetes. Although relatively safe in weak solution, hydroquinone alone or in strong solution is highly toxic and may also give rise to dermatitis and inflammation of the mucous membranes.

Hydrosulphite $(Na_2S_2O_4)$

A term loosely used to denote sodium dithionite or hydrosulphite, a reducing agent, very soluble in water. It is employed as an 0.4 per cent solution in museum-mounting techniques (as an alternative to alcohol), for the restoration of colour in the Kaiserling techniques.

Hypnotics

Organic compounds of this group are sometimes called for in neuropathological techniques where they behave as accentuators (q.v.). Cajal gave them the special designation of accelerators. Chloral hydrate is the most widely used, but veronal, sulphonal and others are used occasionally.

69

I

Impregnation

(1) The process whereby tissues are imbued with a fluid medium such as celloidin, gelatin, or various waxes or resins which, when solidified, offer a supporting matrix to the tissues, so that they may be more easily sectioned.

(2) That group of techniques which, in contradistinction to staining, have as their basic principle the deposition on certain tissue elements of an opaque particulate metallic residue, usually of gold or silver (or their compounds). Their application is considerable and includes the demonstration of such diverse tissue constituents and inclusions as reticulin, melanin and other products of cell metabolism, calcium, spirochaetes, and a wide range of nervous tissue components.

Inclusion bodies

In its wider sense, the term may be applied to any substance, especially of extraneous origin, included within the confines of a nucleus or its cytoplasm. Histologically, its meaning has become differentiated to indicate those intracellular bodies formed as a result of virus activity. Their location within the cell and their staining reactions vary according to the nature of the virus; most nuclear inclusions are acidophil, whilst those occurring in the cytoplasm may contain basophil, acidophil, or mixed elements. These factors influence the choice of method of demonstration. Among the most widely used techniques are Mann's eosin-methyl blue, Lendrum's phloxine-tartrazine, Macchiavello's basic fuchsin-methylene blue, and the Romanovsky stains.

Indirect staining

See Mordants.

Injection methods

This group of techniques is suitable for the study of any intra-luminal system in either microscopic or gross specimens, but is usually applied to the circulatory or respiratory tracts. Its principle depends upon the irrigation of the vessels with normal physiological saline, followed by perfusion under pressure with a semi-solid colloidal mass. Various substances have been utilized for the purpose, including gelatin, celloidin, latex rubber, and some resins. The media employed are often coloured, sometimes differentially, for instance, blue and red to indicate venous and arterial systems. These media, gelatin excepted, are principally designed for use with gross specimens. The surrounding tissues, after hardening of the injection mass, are then cleared or macerated and the ramifying structures thus visualized. Frozen sections may be prepared either from coloured gelatin-injected material, or perhaps better by Fischer's method which uses milk or lard as the injection mass, followed by staining with a fat-soluble dye such as Sudan III or Sudan black.

Intestine

That part of the alimentary tract lying between the pyloric sphincter of the stomach and the anal orifice, consisting of the duodenum, jejunum and ileum which together form the small intestine, and the caecum, colon and rectum, constituting the large intestine. The ileo-caecal valve, to which is attached the appendix vermiformis (q.v.) is found at the junction of the small and large intestines. Histologically the wall of the intestine is composed of diverse tissues, predominantly involuntary muscle and connective tissues, interspersed with nerve plexuses and lined throughout by columnar epithelium. Extending through the whole of both small and large intestines are simple structures like test tubes known as the crypts of Lieberkühn. They alternate, in the small intestine only, with finger-like epithelial projections known as villi. There are four types of constituent cells of the epithelium: (1) a simple columnar cell with a striated border; (2) mucus-secreting (goblet) cells (q.v.); (3) argentaffin (or enterochromaffin) cells (q.v.); and (4) the Paneth cells (q.v.) of the small intestine. Methods for the selective demonstration of 2, 3, and 4, may be found under the appropriate headings.

Intravital staining

That section of vital staining concerned with the colouring of living cells within the body, and confined mostly to the reticulo-endothelial system. It involves the injection into the organism of a colloidal solution of certain dyes such as trypan blue, particles of the dye being ingested by phagocytic cells. After death, the appropriate tissues may be processed and sectioned in the usual way, the dye particles being clearly visible in a suitably counterstained preparation. *See also* Supravital staining.

Iodine

One of the four halogen elements, existing in the form of blue-black scales with a metallic sheen. Its pungent, corrosive vapour is irritant and poisonous. Sparingly soluble in water it dissolves readily in alcohol and in aqueous solutions of iodides. Histologically it has numerous uses: (1) as a mordant in bacterial stains of the Gram group and as part of the Mallory bleach sequence; (2) for the removal of precipitates of mercury following sublimate fixation; (3) for the demonstration, somewhat unspecifically, of amyloid and of glycogen

71

(starch, corpora amylacea and other substances also give a positive reaction); (4) as a constituent of Verhoeff's elastic stain; (5) in Stein's method for bile pigments (q.v.); and (6) for the study of certain hormones and proteins by autoradiographic techniques, in which the ability of radioactive isotopes of iodine (notably I^{131}) to reduce silver is utilized.

Iodine green

A basic dye of the phenyl methane group, occasionally employed as a chromatin stain but more often for the demonstration of amyloid, which it colours metachromatically red.

Iodine green

Ion-exchange resins

See Decalcification.

Iron pigment

See Haemosiderin.

Islets of Langerhans

Small masses of polyhedral or rounded cells lying among the pancreatic acini and demarcated from them by a thin reticular membrane. They are most numerous in the tail of the pancreas. They form the endocrine moiety of the organ, each of their three constituent cell types being responsible for the secretion of a polypeptide hormone. They are members of the APUD series of peripheral neuroendocrine polypeptide-secreting cells, their designation currently being somewhat controversial. Hitherto they have been referred to as alpha, beta and delta cells, secreting respectively glucagon, insulin and gastrin, but a strong body of opinion suggests that the delta cells are essentially variants of the alpha cells and advocates the terms α_2 for alpha (glucagon), β for beta (insulin) and α_1 for delta cells (gastrin).

Methods for the differential demonstration of islet-cell granules include the Masson trichrome stain (and numerous variants), Gomori's aldehyde fuchsin-orange G-light green, and silver impregnation techniques.

Isopropanol (Isopropyl alcohol – $CH_3.CHOH.CH_3$)

An increasingly popular and cheaper alternative to ethyl alcohol for the dehydration of tissues. It is also used as a solvent for fat stains, particularly oil red O.

Isotopes

Chemical elements normally consist of atomic nuclei made up of positively-charged protons and accompanying neutrons of similar mass, the latter possessing no electrical charge. Around these revolve negatively-charged electrons of very small mass (about 1/1,840 of that of the proton). The atomic number of an element represents the number of protons (or electrons); the atomic weight is obtained by the sum of protons and neutrons. In many elements (e.g. oxygen, nitrogen, helium, carbon) the number of protons and neutrons is equal. It would appear therefore that the atomic weights of all elements should be whole numbers, but in a few cases this is not so. Chlorine, for example, has an atomic number of 17 and an atomic weight of 35.5. This is explained by the fact that two types of chlorine exist naturally, differing not in their chemical properties, but in the number of neutrons that each atom possesses. These variants are called isotopes. The first of these, chlorine 35, contains 17 protons and 18 neutrons, the second chlorine 37, has 17 protons and 20 neutrons, each of course with its attendant 17 electrons. These two forms exist in nature in the proportion of 3:1; hence the atomic weight of chlorine is 35.5.

J

Janus green B

A basic azo dye with an associated chromophore, best known as a vital stain, often used in conjunction with neutral red.

Janus green B

Solubility at 20°C is 5.0 per cent in water and 1.0 per cent in alcohol.

K

Kaiserling, Karl (1869–1942)

A German pathologist, noted for his contributions in the field of medical museum technology. The preservative solutions and methods he devised are still in current use in many laboratories, and entail fixation in a formalin solution buffered with potassium acetate and potassium nitrate, followed by treatment in 80—90 per cent alcohol to restore the natural colours. Mounting is effected in a preservative solution of glycerine and potassium acetate.

Kephalin

See Cephalin.

Kerasin

One of the three cerebrosides or glycolipids so far established (the others being phrenosin and nervon). On hydrolysis all cerebrosides yield a fatty acid, a carbohydrate, and the nitrogenous base sphingosine. The fatty acid characteristic of kerasin is lignoceric acid, $C_{23}H_{47}COOH$.

Pathologically the lipidosis known as Gaucher's disease is characterized by an excessive accumulation of kerasin.

Keratin

A substance occurring in skin, hair, nails, horn etc., constituting, together with collagen, elastin, and ossein, the group of fibrous proteins, or scleroproteins which form most of the supporting and protective structures of the body. It differs from them in possessing a high sulphur content mainly in the form of the amino acid, cystine. It resists solution in trypsin and pepsin but is attacked by alkali sulphides, which fact is utilized in the preparation of depilatories. Its histological demonstration may be effected with Gram's crystal violet, or Heidenhain's haematoxylin, or more specifically with peracetic acid-azure eosin.

Ketosteroids

A group of steroids of considerable biological importance, in which a ketonic oxygen is attached to a carbon atom at the 3 or 17 position in the characteristic steroid cyclopentophenanthrene structure.

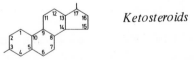

Ketosteroids

The group includes the corticosteroids and the sex hormones, testosterone and progesterone, having their ketonic group at the 3 position, and androsterone and oestrone at the 17 position. Their histochemical demonstration is fraught with difficulties; several methods have been devised but none of indisputable specificity up to the present time.

Kidneys

Bilateral bean-shaped organs lying one on each side of the lumbar spine, they are compound tubular glands invested with a fibrous capsule. The organs are divided into a cortex, lying below the capsule, and a medulla adjacent to the renal pelvis. The functional unit is the nephron, of which each kidney contains at least one million, composed of a tuft of minute capillaries, known as a glomerulus, invested in a delicate fibrous capsule (Bowman's capsule) and continuous with the renal tubules, the whole minute organ acting as a filter. The kidneys control the concentration of the blood constituents by filtration, excretion and re-absorption of fluid, and also the end-products of nitrogen metabolism and the electrolytes contained therein. Staining techniques that may be applied especially to the kidney include: (1) for general histology, the Masson's trichrome group, techniques for elastic fibres, and the PAS methods; and (2) for special cytology, methods for haemoglobin and other pigments, vital staining and injection procedures, mitochondrial stains, and various techniques for the demonstration of such products as amyloid, calcium, lipids, etc.

Kóssa, Julius von Magyary

A Hungarian physician whose test for calcium salts in tissue sections is a universally-employed technique. It entails impregnation in silver nitrate with the formation of silver phosphate or carbonate at the sites of the corresponding calcium salts, with subsequent reduction to black metallic silver either by exposure to ultra-violet light or by the use of photographic developers.

See also Calcium.

Kultchitsky, Nicolai (1856–1925)

A Russian anatomist who gave his name first to the argentaffin (q.v.) or enterochromaffin cells of the intestine; secondly to a haematoxylin solution used widely in a technique for the demonstration of myelin.

Kupffer cells

Phagocytic reticulo-endothelial cells lining the sinusoids of the liver. They may be demonstrated intra-vitally by injection of the organism with such dyes as trypan blue and Indian ink.

Kurloff bodies

Cytoplasmic inclusions of unknown origin, found commonly in the mononuclear leucocytes of guinea-pigs and other mammals. They are PAS positive and strongly phloxinophil.

L

Lakes

Dye lakes are coloured compounds, usually insoluble in water,
and formed by the interaction of dye and mordant, which may
attach themselves to certain tissue elements. They are soluble in
excess of the mordant used, and in acidic solutions.

Lapping compounds

See Abrasive powder.

Lead

The recognition in tissues of lead compounds is occasionally
required, there being several methods available for their detection.
Fresh unripened haematoxylin is suggested by Mallory, while
Frankenberger and Crétin advise acidified potassium chromate, the
lead salts being converted into yellow lead chromate. Perhaps the
most reliable method is that of Feigl using salts of rhodizonic acid,
which give coloured precipitates with such diverse elements as
barium, bismuth, cadmium, calcium, lead, mercury, silver,
strontium, thallium, tin, uranium, and zinc. The technique may be
rendered entirely specific by prior treatment with weak sulphuric
acid.

Lecithins

The most important of the phospholipids (q.v.) and an essential
constituent of all living cells. On hydrolysis they produce fatty acids,
glycerol, phosphoric acid, and the nitrogenous base choline.

Lecithins

For their histological demonstration *see* Phospholipids.

Leprosy

Histologically the demonstration of *Mycobacterium leprae* may
be effected by the Ziehl-Neelsen method, with careful differentiation
in weak acid. A better method is the Wade-Fite method, whose basic
principle is similar but which has the advantage of restoring acid-
fastness by the replacement of xylene as a decerating agent with a
turpentine-paraffin oil mixture.

Leuckhart's moulds

L-shaped pieces of metal, usually brass, of varying sizes, used in pairs in conjunction with a flat glass or metal base for the casting or embedding of tissues in paraffin wax.

Leuco-dyes

A series of colourless compounds resulting from the reduction of certain dyes, whereby the chromophoric groups are destroyed. This process may occur in several ways: for example, the NO_2 (nitro) chromophore may be reduced to the NH_2 (amino) group; the quinoid linkage may be broken and hydrogen atoms become attached to the free valencies; or the acid radicle may in certain cases be removed to form a pseudo-base or carbinol again lacking a chromophoric group. Restoration of the colour may usually be achieved by a reversal of the decolourization process or by some associated method. Thus acid fuchsin and dyes of the phenolphthalein group utilize this property and constitute valuable acid-base indicators. Basic fuchsin may be used for the detection of aldehydes (Schiff reagent); and patent blue and similar dyes for the demonstration of peroxidase activity. The principle may be extended to embrace a long list of dyes which can form the basis for Schiff-type reagents; most of these can be dismissed on the score of instability or poor colour values. A fluorescent Schiff utilizing acriflavine hydrochloride in place of basic fuchsin has been employed for the demonstration of DNA, mucin and basement membranes.

Levaditi, Constantin (1874–1953)

A Rumanian bacteriologist, noted especially in histological circles for his block impregnation method for the demonstration of spirochaetes in tissues. The technique entails fixation in formalin, followed by treatment with 1.5 per cent silver nitrate, and subsequent reduction in pyrogallic acid-formalin.

Leydig cells

These interstitial testicular cells are characterized by the presence of lipofuscin.

See Lipofuscin, for methods of demonstration.

Light green FS

An acid dye of the phenyl-methane group, widely used as a counterstain to haematoxylin or safranin, and in the PAS and trichrome variants. It is a constituent also of Twort's compound stain for micro-organisms and of the Papanicolaou cytological stain.

It is prone to fading in bright sunlight, and for this reason Fast green FCF may be preferred.

Light green FS

Solubility at 20°C is 20 per cent in water and 0.75 per cent in alcohol.

Lipase

The lipases form a subdivision of the enzyme group known as the aliesterases, and are capable of hydrolysing glycerol esters of long-chain fatty acids (the simple lipids). Their most common site is the pancreas. Their power to hydrolyse fatty acid esters is utilized in their demonstration by the 'Tween' methods, the Tweens being water-soluble esters of such acids saturated or unsaturated, with polyglycols, in the presence of calcium salts. Calcium soaps are deposited at the site of enzyme activity, these being converted by treatment with lead nitrate into lead soaps. These in turn react with ammonium sulphide to form brown lead sulphide. Other methods include the indoxyl acetate method of Barrnett and Seligman, resulting in the production of indigo, and the coupling azo-dye method of Nachlas and Seligman.

See also Aliesterases; Tweens.

Lipid

This has become the generally accepted term to denote any naturally-occurring fatty substance, insoluble in water and soluble in so called 'fat solvents' such as benzene, ether, chloroform, etc. The designation 'lipoid' has little to commend it and might well be abandoned, whilst 'lipin' or 'lipine', if used at all, should be restricted to indicate the compound lipids, namely the phospholipids and the cerebrosides.

Lipin or Lipine

See Lipid.

Lipofuscins

A group of pigments, arising from the oxidation of certain lipids and lipoproteins, occurring in such diverse sites as myocardium, liver, adrenals, testes and ganglion cells, in the first of which it is often referred to as brown atrophy or 'wear-and-tear' pigment. The histological reactions of these yellowish-brown granular pigments are

78

largely dependent on their degree of oxidation. They are invariably iron-negative, and in the less oxidized forms are sudanophil and slightly basophil. The degree of pigmentation increases with oxidation, associated with concomitant loss of sudanophilia, and an increase of basophilia, together with an ability to reduce Schmorl's ferric chloride-ferricyanide and ammoniacal silver solutions. Furthermore, most of the partially oxidized lipofuscins are actively fluorescent, acid-fast, and PAS positive.

Liver

The largest gland of the body, reddish-brown, roughly pyramidal, and occupying the upper part of the right side of the abdominal cavity. It has numerous functions: (1) it is concerned with metabolism of fats, amino-acids and carbohydrates; (2) it acts as a store-house for glycogen, hormones, enzymes and vitamins, and plays a part in the regulation of the blood sugar; (3) it is responsible for the synthesis of prothrombin, heparin, fibrinogen and plasma proteins; (4) it destroys broken-down red blood corpuscles from which the bile pigments are continuously elaborated and transferred for storage to the adjacent gall bladder; and (5) it is the body's most important centre for the detoxication of unwanted substances.

See also Kupffer cells; Bile canaliculi.

Lugol, Jean Guillaume Auguste (1786—1851)

A French physician who has given his name to a wide range of iodine-potassium iodide solutions, that nowadays generally consist of iodine 1.0 g, potassium iodide 2.0 g, and distilled water 100.0 ml. It is called for in several techniques: for instance, for the removal of mercury precipitates from tissues; as an integral stage of the Mallory bleach (q.v.); for the demonstration of amyloid and glycogen; and in some of the Gram stain variants for micro-organisms.

Lungs

Paired respiratory organs occupying the major part of the thoracic cavity, the right consisting of three lobes, the left of two. They are closely invested by smooth glistening serous membranes, the pleurae, and have a spongy consistency being composed of innumerable air-sacs or alveoli. The main function of the lungs is to assimilate oxygen from the air by inspiration and to diffuse it through the alveolar walls into the blood stream, from which carbon dioxide is removed and expelled by expiration.

Luxol fast blue

A basic dye of the copper phthalocyanin (CuPC) series, closely related to the Alcian blue group, but solubilized by sulphonic acid derivatives instead of chloromethyl groups. It is an excellent stain for myelin on frozen, paraffin, or celloidin sections. The staining mechanism is somewhat obscure but it seems likely that the lipoproteins are the reactive constituents. Neutral red has been employed as a counterstain, but cresyl fast (echt) violet is probably preferable, each of these stains forming an intensely coloured complex with the Luxol fast blue in the myelinated areas. Nissl substance is moreover effectively demonstrated by each of these counterstains.

See also Alcian blue.

LVN (low viscosity nitrocellulose)

This embedding medium is an alternative to celloidin, and by virtue of its lower viscosity permits a higher concentration to be used with greater speed of infiltration. Harder blocks and therefore thinner sections may be obtained, but they are more liable to crack than corresponding celloidin sections. This fault may to some extent be obviated by incorporating 1.0 per cent tricresyl phosphate or 0.5 per cent castor oil in the embedding medium.

See also Celloidin.

Lymph nodes

Aggregations of lymphatic tissue to form distinct encapsulated organs lying along the course of lymphatic vessels. Their functions include filtration of the lymph and the elimination of toxins and other foreign material from it; and the manufacture of lymphocytes which are added to the lymph passing through the nodes.

Lysosome

A minute cytoplasmic inclusion resembling a mitochrondrion in appearance, but smaller, somewhat denser, and lacking the characteristic cristae of mitochondria. It is rich in enzymes, notably acid phosphatase, and rupture of its membrane may well be responsible for cell autolysis.

M

Maceration

In histology, the immersion of solid tissue in a fluid in order to promote dissolution of the softer elements. It is used especially in the demonstration of bone lesions for museum purposes and may be achieved in several ways, the choice being governed largely by the nature of the lesion. The most effective methods, and equally the most nauseating, are by 'putrefaction', either spontaneous or expedited by the additionof proteolytic bacteria. More rapidly, maceration may be effected by boiling or autoclaving the specimen with dilute caustic soda.

Macroglia

A term sometimes used to denote neuroglial cells of ectodermal origin, namely the astrocytes, both fibrous and protoplasmic, and oligodendrocytes, but excluding the microglia, which are of mesodermal origin.

Macrophages (Gk *makros,* large + *phagein,* to eat)

Large phagocytic cells present normally in connective tissue and in various organs such as lung, liver, spleen and lymph glands, and pathologically in areas of inflammation. They readily ingest particles of dye *in vivo* from colloidal solutions and hence may be demonstrated intravitally by such agents as trypan blue, Indian ink, etc.

Macroscopic

Visible to the naked eye, without recourse to microscopy.

Magenta

A name sometimes given to the pararosanilins of the phenylmethane family; acid magenta and basic magenta are more often referred to as acid and basic fuchsin (q.v.) respectively.

Magnification

The apparent increase in the size of an object when viewed through a single or multiple lens system as in a microscope; the ratio of apparent to actual linear dimensions. Most modern oculars and objectives are engraved with their magnifying powers.

Malarial pigment (haemozoin)

A haematogenous dark brown, intracellular, particulate pigment, present in the malarial parasite and affected red blood corpuscles, and in phagocytes adjacent to blood vessels. It is similar, if not chemically identical to formalin pigment (acid formaldehyde haematin, q.v.), being readily soluble in alkaline alcohol and in saturated alcoholic picric acid.

Malignant

A term applied to various diseases, but especially to neoplasms or new-growths, denoting a virulence of such degree as to constitute a threat to life and a tendency to recur even after total extirpation. *See also* Benign.

Malignant cells

In exfoliative cytological material, malignant cells may be seen to exhibit certain abnormal features, especially of the cell nucleus. The criteria most generally accepted are: (1) nuclear enlargement and a

consequent disturbance of the normal nucleus/cytoplasm ratio;
(2) irregularity of nuclear outline and variability in their size and
shape, lobulation being a common characteristic; and (3) uneven
distribution and clumping of chromatin particles, this often leading
to hyperchromasia. Multinucleation and multinucleolation may also
occur.

For the cytological demonstration of malignant cells *see*
Papanicolaou; Exfoliative cytology.

Mallory, Frank Burr (1862–1941)

An American pathologist who devised numerous staining methods,
with particular emphasis on connective and nervous tissues. In the
former group his method utilizing aniline blue, orange G and acid
fuchsin is the best known, and in the latter, phosphotungstic acid-
haematoxylin. He also introduced a mordanting sequence known as
the 'Mallory bleach', whereby sections are treated successively with
iodine, sodium thiosulphate, potassium permanganate and oxalic
acid. This procedure is often employed as a prelude to trichrome and
phosphotungstic acid haematoxylin staining following sublimate or
dichromate fixation or post-chroming.

Mann, Gustav (1864–1921)

A German physiologist, much of whose work was done in Oxford.
His *Physiological Histology,* published in 1902, is still regarded as a
classic. From the practical viewpoint his most valuable contribution
to the repertoire was his eosin-methyl blue method which, apart
from its uses as a general stain, had especial value for such diverse
elements as nerve cells, the chromophil cells of the pituitary and
Negri bodies.

Marchi, Vittorio (1851–1908)

An Italian physician remembered for his method for degenerating
myelin. The technique depends on the fact that, whereas all lipids
are capable of reducing osmium tetroxide to its lower black oxide,
this property is inhibited in the case of the compound lipids of
which normal myelin is largely composed, by treatment with
potassium dichromate, which is itself an oxidizing agent. Degenerating myelin, however, is rich in unsaturated fatty acids such as oleic
acid. These remain unoxidized by the dichromate but are nevertheless susceptible to oxidation by osmium tetroxide which is thereby
reduced to form the black oxide.

Martius yellow

An acid dye of the nitro group, of particular use in the trichrome
techniques and in methods for fibrin. Its formula and its reactions
resemble those of picric acid.

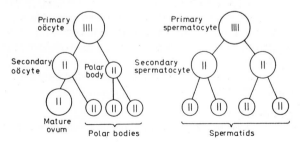

Martius yellow

Solubility at 20°C is 4.5 per cent in water and 0.15 per cent in alcohol.

Mayer, Paul (1848–1923)

A German histologist remembered for his invaluable contribution to stain techniques. Among the solutions he devised were his haemalum, a widely-used nuclear stain, and several recipes utilizing carmine, in particular mucicarmine (q.v.) for the demonstration of mucin.

Meiosis

Heterotypical cellular division, occurring only during maturation of the sex cells (gametogenesis). It is sometimes referred to as reduction division and results in the production of haploid cells from diploid parent cells. In the female, the immature ovum or primary oocyte increases in size and then undergoes first heterotypical division into a secondary oocyte and a polar body, each containing half the number of chromosomes characteristic of the species (23 in man: 22 somatic and 1 sex chromosome). Further division of the secondary oocyte follows, this time without reduction of the chromosomal number, giving rise to the mature ovum together with a second polar body. The original polar body may also divide to produce two further similar bodies, making three in all. These are incapable of further development and are in fact abortive ova. In the male an analogous process occurs, the primary spermatocyte giving rise to two secondary spermatocytes with halved chromosomal complement. These in turn divide to form four spermatids of equal size and potential. Thus when spermatozoon and mature ovum unite in the process of fertilization the total complement of chromosomes is restored in man to 44 autosomes and 2 sex chromosomes.

Melanin (Gk *melas,* black)

An endogenous pigment occurring normally in hair, the basal layer of the epidermis, the eye, the brain stem, etc. Pathologically it may be found in tumours, both benign and malignant, ranging from small moles in the skin to the metastasising malignant melanomas, and in Addison's disease. It increases also in white skin when it is exposed to ultraviolet light and may be manifested as suntan or as freckles. The term melanin is something of a misnomer as the natural colour of the pigment may range from yellow through brown to black, the amount of pigment being responsible for the colour variation in the skins of different races. Its exact chemical composition is uncertain but it is thought to be a derivative of tyrosine.

It resists solution in most chemicals, including strong acids and fat solvents, but dissolves in concentrated alkaline solutions. Histologically its demonstration may be effected by impregnation with ammoniacal silver (Fontana's method), by the reduction of Schmorl's reagent (q.v.), or negatively by its ability to be bleached by oxidizing agents such as hydrogen peroxide (a property well recognized by 'bottle-blondes'), nascent chlorine, potassium permanganate-oxalic acid, and borax-ferricyanide.

See also Tyrosinase.

Mercuric chloride ($HgCl_2$)

This heavy white compound, popularly known as corrosive sublimate, is a virulent poison, either by absorption through the skin or more rapidly by swallowing or inhalation of the dust. Most metals, especially aluminium, are attacked by it. It has a wide range of uses in the histology laboratory: (1) as a fixative, usually in combination with other fixing agents such as formalin, alcohol, or potassium dichromate; (2) for the impregnation of Golgi apparatus (with potassium dichromate) and of astrocytes (with gold chloride); (3) as a mordant prior to Mallory's phosphotungstic acid-haematoxylin and the trichrome techniques, and in the Hoyer thionin method for mucins; and (4) in the plasmal reaction for acetal lipids from which aldehydes are liberated by hydrolysis with mercuric chloride. One of its disadvantages, apart from its toxicity, is that when used as a fixative an amorphous greyish-black precipitate is deposited in the tissues. This may be removed from the tissue block by adding a little alcoholic iodine to the 70 per cent alcohol during dehydration, or by treatment of the cut sections with iodine solution prior to staining.

Mercuric oxide (HgO)

The two forms of this compound, red and yellow, are chemically identical, the former existing as crystalline powder or scales, the latter as a fine powder. This finely powdered yellow form is used histologically as an oxidizing agent for haematoxylin solutions, e.g. Harris's formula. It should be protected from light and is highly poisonous.

Metanil yellow

An acid dye of the mono-azo group, used occasionally as a plasma stain in contrast, for example, to haematoxylin and acid fuchsin or to stains such as crystal violet and mucicarmine.

Metanil yellow

Solubility at $20^\circ C$ is 5.3 per cent in water and 1.45 per cent in alcohol.

Metaphase

The second of the four phases of mitosis (q.v.) or cell division, it follows prophase and is characterized by the arrangement of the chromosomes in the equatorial region of the achromatic spindle, the centrioles having moved to its opposite ends. The stage is completed by longitudinal division of each of the chromosomes into two chromatids.

Methacrylate

See Acrylic resins.

Methasol fast blue

A member of the copper phthalocyanin (CuPC) group of dyes, its behaviour is essentially similar to that of Luxol fast blue (q.v.).

Methylation

One of the most important of the 'blocking' techniques. The characteristic staining reactions of both sulphated and acid mucopolysaccharides may be blocked by treatment with methyl alcohol (CH_3OH). In the former group a soluble acid methyl sulphate is formed, leaving behind the unsulphated polysaccharide. In the latter, esterification of the carboxylic acid or other acidic groups takes place. In each case loss of characteristic staining occurs, but this may be restored in the case of the acidic compounds by saponification with potassium hydroxide. A similar procedure may be employed in the demonstration of carboxylic acid-containing lipids.

See also Blocking.

Methyl blue

A strongly acid dye of the phenylmethane group, not to be confused with the basic dye methylene blue. It may be used instead of aniline blue WS as a connective tissue stain, or with eosin, as in Mann's method which is of particular use in the demonstration of protozoa and virus inclusions.

Methyl blue

Solubility at $20°C$ is 10.0 per cent in water.

Methylene blue

An important basic dye of the thiazin subgroup of quinone-imine compounds. Histologically it is a very useful nuclear stain, especially in contrast to red stains, e.g. Ziehl-Neelsen's method for acid-fast bacilli and Macchiavallo's inclusion body technique. It is also called for in Ehrlich's method for the supra-vital demonstration of peripheral nerve endings. Perhaps, however, its most valuable application is in the realm of the Romanovsky stains, where it is used in combination with eosin to form the neutral stains of Leishman, Wright, etc. The efficacy of this group is enhanced by the ability of methylene blue to 'polychrome' or oxidize to form lower homologues of the thiazin group such as the azures (q.v.). This phenomenon occurs spontaneously both with the dry powder and in alcoholic or watery solutions, but more readily in alkaline solution or at higher temperatures. The resultant mixture of methylene blue with its lower (more violet) homologues is known as polychrome methylene blue, and affords a much wider tinctorial range.

Methylene blue

Solubility at $20°C$ is 2.0 per cent in water and 1.6 per cent in alcohol.

Methyl green

A basic dye of the phenylmethane group, heptamethyl pararosanilin, differing only from crystal violet by the presence of an additional methyl group. It has certain metachromatic properties but its greatest value is as a chromatin stain. The Unna-Pappenheim method calls for it in combination with pyronin, which stains the RNA red in contrast to the green of the DNA. In dry form it tends to break down into crystal violet, some of which is normally present in the commercial sample. This may be removed by washing in chloroform in which the violet dye is readily soluble.

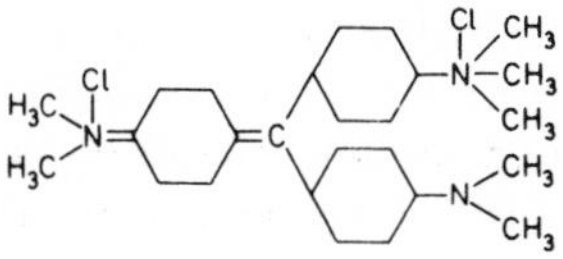

Methyl green

Solubility at $20°C$ is 8.0 per cent in water.

Methyl violet

A basic dye, or mixture of similar dyes, of the phenylmethane group. It is normally available as a mixture of crystal violet (hexamethyl pararosanilin) and its lower homologues (tetra- and pentamethyl pararosanilins) and its uses are similar to those of crystal violet.

The formula for the tetra compound is:

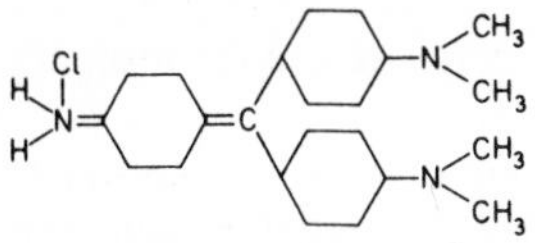

Methyl violet

Solubility at $20°C$ is 5.0 per cent in water and 5.0 per cent in alcohol.

Microglia

A subgroup of neuroglial cells arising from the mesoderm, phagocytic in nature, and forming part of the reticulo-endothelial system. They are absent at birth and invade the brain after 3–4 weeks from the pia. They have a small elongated, triangular or navicular nucleus, scanty cytoplasm, and several branching twig-like processes. They may be found in the white matter but are much more numerous in the grey. In certain pathological conditions they may proliferate and assume bizarre shapes, e.g. in epilepsy and inflammatory lesions. Although their nuclei may be seen in routine stains, the processes can only be observed after metallic impregnation by such methods as Hortega, Penfield, and Weil-Davenport, preferably on frozen sections.

See also Neuroglia; Oligodendroglia.

87

Micro-incineration

In histology, the analysis and identification of inorganic matter by subjecting tissue sections to high temperatures (600–650°C), thereby destroying organic material and leaving behind the mineral salts *in situ*. These may be examined microscopically by fluorescence, polariscopy, dark-ground illumination or oblique light, or they may undergo chemical analysis. Difficulties of interpretation are, however, considerable and the technique itself is by no means easy; care must be taken, for example, that fixation and processing are such that no extraneous inorganic matter (e.g. sodium chloride or mercuric chloride) be introduced, and that the mineral content already present in the tissues should not be appreciably reduced. Fixation in formol-alcohol and freeze-drying have each been recommended. Furthermore, the temperature must be controlled carefully; too rapid an increase causes dislocation of the mineralized areas. A muffle furnace using quartz slides is usually employed, but a much simpler and more economic method has recently been devised by Swettenham; the sections, mounted on glass slides, are placed on a heavy iron base plate; heating is carried out by two Bunsen burners, and the incineration temperature is confirmed by placing a few crystals of cuprous iodide (this melts at 605°C) on one slide. The use of glass rather than quartz slides has a further advantage in that they soften slightly at this temperature and the inorganic salts become bound to the glass. Hence, after cooling, preparations may be mounted permanently in balsam or plastic mountants without noticeable disturbance. Control slides of parallel unincinerated sections should always be used for comparison.

Micrometre

Equivalent to a millionth part (10^{-6}) of a metre, or 10,000 Å, usually represented by the symbol μm, and the standard unit of measurement in micrometry and in microtomy. It is roughly equal to 1/25,400 of an inch. Formerly this unit was known as the micron (μ), but in conformity with the Système International, the term has been replaced by 'micrometre'.

Micrometry

The measurement of very small objects in terms of micrometres, the micrometre (μm) being the unit of length in light microscopy and equivalent to 0.001 mm. Such estimations may be carried out with the aid of two micrometer scales, an eyepiece micrometer resting on the field stop of the ocular, and a stage micrometer on the stage of the microscope. The eyepiece micrometer is a disc engraved with an arbitrary scale divided usually into 100 equal divisions. The stage micrometer consists of a 3 in X 1 in slide on which a millimetre scale is engraved in 1/10 and 1/100 graduations. By calibration of the eyepiece scale against that of the stage micrometer scale, the absolute value of each division of the former may be determined. The stage micrometer may then be replaced by the test object and the required direct measurement effected. Other scales having a known calibration such as a standard haemacytometer may serve as a substitute for the stage micrometer. An alternative method sometimes used for multiple measurements within the same field is that of projection on to a screen of the stage micrometer, the divisions of which may be measured on the screen with a centimetre rule and the magnification calculated. The test object is then projected and its measurement noted.

Micron
See Micrometre.

Micro-organisms
Histologically their demonstration is dealt with under the appropriate separate headings.

See Gram; Negri bodies; Inclusion bodies; Levaditi; Fungi; Leprosy; Ziehl-Neelsen.

Microtome
An instrument for cutting sections of tissue of uniform even thickness for examination under the microscope. Several types have been devised, each with its own modifications, the choice of instrument being to some extent governed by the tissue- or cell-components subsequently to be demonstrated.

(1) The base sledge microtome, a heavy stable machine with a fixed knife; the block is attached to a sliding unit and moves backwards and forwards against the knife edge. This instrument is normally used for paraffin-embedded material but may be adapted for use with celloidin-embedded or frozen tissues; because of its size and stability it will permit large blocks to be cut.

(2) The sliding microtome in which the knife moves horizontally towards a fixed block which is raised after each section has been cut by advancement along an inclined plane. This machine is best suited to celloidin material, but again may be used for paraffin sectioning.

(3) The rotary microtome, so called because actuation is achieved by rotation of the hand-wheel. The block moves vertically up and down a steel groove, its advancement being controlled by means of a micrometer screw. This instrument is suited to paraffin blocks and is recommended for serial sectioning.

(4)   The rocking microtome or 'rocker', in which the block is attached to the end of a lever and moves in an arc against a fixed knife, and may be advanced by a micrometer screw. This microtome is again suitable for paraffin blocks, preferably small, and may be used for serial work. It is occasionally employed for celloidin material.

(5)   The freezing microtome, an apparatus which incorporates a device for freezing the tissue by means of compressed carbon dioxide or ethyl chloride, or by a thermomodule (q.v.). Here the knife pivots through a horizontal arc against an immobile block, which is raised by a micrometer screw.

See also Cryostat; Ultra-microtome.

Microtome knives

These are classified according to their cross-section into (1) bi-plane or wedge, (2) plane-concave, and (3) bi-concave or hollow-ground. It is claimed by the more dogmatic authorities that each of these has its own specific and exclusive use; there is in fact considerable latitude in the utilization of each type, any one of them, provided of course it is sharp, being suitable for paraffin or frozen cutting; the only reservation is perhaps that a plane-concave knife with a pronounced concavity is more suited to celloidin work. Specially prepared knives made from hardened alloys are available for cutting very tough material, e.g. undecalcified bone.

See also Heiffor knife; Ultra-microtome.

Microtomy (Gk *micros,* small + *temnein,* to cut)

The process of cutting thin sections of tissue for microscopic examination. The term usually embraces the techniques of section-cutting with or without recourse to embedding media, and the use and maintenance of the microtomes and accessories (knives, hones and strops) concerned.

Mitochondria (Gk *mitos,* a thread + *chondrion,* a granule)

A normal cytoplasmic component of all living cells; mitochondria may exist in the form of spherical, rod-shaped, or filamentous bodies ($0.5-1.0$ μm in diameter and up to 7.0 μm long), containing predominantly nucleoproteins and phospholipids. Their function appears to be concerned with cell respiration and enzymatic activity. They may vary in size, number and shape from one cell type to another but are extremely numerous in most cell types (e.g. 2,500 in a liver cell). They are rapidly autolysed and are among the first structures to disappear after the death of the cell. Prompt fixation is therefore essential, Zenker-formol followed by post-chroming probably being the most satisfactory process. Acetic acid causes destruction or distortion of mitochondria and should be avoided. They can be demonstrated in fresh tissue by vital stains such as Janus green, or in paraffin sections by Altmann's aniline—acid fuchsin; by the Champy-Kull acid fuchsin—toluidine blue—aurantia sequence; by Heidenhain's iron alum—haematoxylin; or by the Millon reagent, which latter method is based on visualization of the tyrosine component of the mitochondrial proteins.

Mitosis

The normal process by which a cell nucleus divides to form two daughter cells, each containing the same number of chromosomes and hereditary characteristics as the parent cell. Mitosis is divided into four stages: prophase, metaphase, anaphase, and telophase, which are treated under their respective headings. Mitotic figures are well seen in preparations stained by Heidenhain's iron alum—haematoxylin, or by Feulgen's technique. The study of mitosis has been considerably facilitated in recent years by the administration of colchicine, which inhibits formation of the achromatic spindle and arrests the process in the metaphase, the chromosomes remaining clumped in the centre of the cell.

Mono-azo

See Azo dyes.

Mordants

Substances which act as intermediaries between stain and tissue, by forming a coloured compound or 'lake' with the stain to which the tissue becomes firmly attached. Such a device is necessary where no direct affinity between stain and tissue exists, the procedure being known as 'indirect staining' (compare with direct staining). The bond thus established may only be broken by solution of the 'lake' in a suitable differentiating fluid, sometimes the mordant itself, sometimes a weak acid solution. The chief mordants used in histology are the alums (q.v.) and salts of ferric iron and aluminium. Mordants may be incorporated in the staining solution, or in the fixative, or may be used as a separate solution prior to staining. Of the common dyes requiring mordants, haematoxylin and carmine are perhaps the most important.

Mounting media

Transparent, colourless or nearly colourless fluids, applied to microscopical preparations, which enable a glass coverslip to be attached to them, thus rendering them more or less permanent and suitable for microscopical study. Such media may be solutions of one or more solids, mixtures of liquids, or single liquid reagents.

91

They should possess some degree of viscosity in order to promote adherence between coverslip and slide, and most media tend to become more viscous and ultimately solidify. The refractive index of mounting media is of considerable importance: in the case of stained paraffin sections, cleared with xylene, maximum visibility is obtained with media whose refractive index approximates to that of the fixed tissue proteins, a transparent optically perfect image thus being obtained. Unstained preparations for examination by phase contrast or by direct microscopy should be mounted in a medium whose refractive index differs slightly from that of the tissue proteins. Some tissue constituents, notably lipids, are soluble in xylene and alcohol and must be mounted from water in a hydrophil mountant, i.e. one that either contains water or is miscible with it, like glycerine. Some confusion is engendered by the use of the term 'mounting media' as applied to the substances, solid or liquid, in which gross specimens are mounted for museum purposes.

See also Resins.

Mucicarmine

A name given by Mayer to a mixture of carmine (q.v.) and aluminium chloride, used for staining mucins. A modification, known as Southgate's mucicarmine, incorporating aluminium hydroxide as well as the chloride, has to some extent superseded the original recipe.

Mucins

A term somewhat lacking in precision used to describe certain tissue substances and embracing a wide range of carbohydrates, including the neutral and acid mucopolysaccharides (q.v.), the mucoproteins (q.v.) and glycoproteins, and the mucolipids (q.v.).

Mucolipids

These are composed of a carbohydrate-fatty acid complex, the most important subgroup being the cerebrosides or galactolipids (q.v.).

Mucopolysaccharides

These carbohydrates may be divided readily into two groups, neutral and acid. The former is found rarely in the higher mammals, its commonest site being the cellulose-like substance, chitin (q.v.). Acid mucopolysaccharides, however, occur widely in such sites as cartilage, umbilical cord, and the mucosa of the alimentary canal. A wide range of techniques may be used to demonstrate the acid mucopolysaccharides, such as PAS, Alcian blue, dialysed iron, and the metachromatic thiazin dyes.

Mucoproteins

A group of polysaccharide-protein compounds, including the glycoproteins and the sialomucins, the classification being dependent on the ratio of polysaccharide to protein, The glycoproteins with a carbohydrate content of less than 4 per cent occur in connective tissues, certain hormones, and in amyloid. They give a positive PAS reaction but are usually negative to toluidine blue and Alcian blue. The mucoproteins react similarly but the sialomucins are usually positive to Alcian blue. Mucoproteins occur in salivary gland tissue and in some gonadotropic hormones.

Müller, Hermann Franz (1886–1898)

A Viennese histologist, who gave his name to a potassium dichromate–sodium sulphate solution used in bone histology. Excellent results may be obtained by prolonged treatment in Müller's fluid (say 6 months) followed by completion of decalcification in weak formic acid and embedding in celloidin; the whole process takes a year or longer and is therefore impractical for urgently needed material.

Muscle

The contractile tissue of the body constituting, with epithelial, connective, and nervous tissues, one of the four basic tissues of the body. It may be subdivided into (1) smooth or involuntary; (2) striated or voluntary (skeletal); and (3) striated involuntary (cardiac) muscle. Differentiation between striated and unstriated muscle may be clearly seen in sections stained by Mallory's phosphotungstic acid–haematoxylin, or by Heidenhain's iron haematoxylin, or by polariscopic examination.

See also Cross striations.

Myelin

A complex substance found in the sheaths of medullated nerve fibres, and responsible for the characteristic appearance of the white matter in the CNS. It is composed largely of lipid material of widely diverse nature, including various phospholipids and sphingolipids, cholesterol and its esters, and a small amount of neutral fat. Some protein is also present and certain enzymes have been identified. The myelin of the central nervous system differs slightly in composition from that of the peripheral nervous system, especially in protein and enzyme content. The oligodendrocytes are responsible for the manufacture of myelin in the central nervous system, and in the peripheral nerves the myelin is laid down by the Schwann cells rotating around the axon.

Numerous methods are available for the positive demonstration of normal myelin, utilizing haematoxylin in particular, most of them based on Weigert's original method. The modifications of Pal, Kultschitsky, and Loyez are probably the most popular. More recently the Luxol fast blue and Solochrome cyanin RS methods (q.v.) have tended to supersede the older techniques.

See also Marchi.

N

Nadi reaction

See Cytochrome oxidase.

Natural dyes

A small but important number of dyes is still obtained from natural sources and has not as yet been superseded by synthetic substitutes. Among the most important are haematoxylin and carmine, and to a lesser degree alizarin and orcein, both of which can nowadays be synthesized. Occasionally such dyes as litmus, indigo and saffron are called for. The most important members of this group are dealt with under the appropriate headings.

Necrosis (Gk *nekros,* dead)

Death of a portion of a tissue, brought about by any one of several factors, including circulatory disturbance, irradiation, or bacterial, chemical, traumatic or toxic action.

Negri bodies

The characteristic cytoplasmic inclusion bodies of rabies, found in the neurones of the central nervous system, especially in the hippocampus. They may be stained with basic fuchsin, as in the Macchiavello method, or by the Giemsa-type methods.

Nerve endings

The terminal arborizations of nerve fibres, either axons or dendrites, arising from the neurones. They may be motor, sensory or secretory and occur in most body tissues, often in intimate contact with another nerve ending to form a synapse. By such a mechanism nerve impulses are transmitted throughout the body. Their demonstration may be effected in several ways. Ideally perhaps they may be studied supra-vitally with methylene blue. Alternative procedures are: block impregnation with such methods as Nonidez, using chloral hydrate followed by silver nitrate impregnation and reduction in pyrogallol-formol; or Ranvier's classical method on teased material, using lemon juice, followed by gold chloride and reduction in formic acid. The Bielschowsky group of methods for neurofibrils sometimes gives favourable results, provided thick sections (30–50 μm) are used.

Neurofibrils

Fine fibres occurring in the cytoplasm of the neurones and extending into their processes, and grouping together in sheaves to form axis cylinders and dendrites. Their demonstration is difficult by routine methods, but may be effected by metallic impregnation in techniques of the Bielschowsky type.

Neuroglia

The general name for those structures that afford support for the nervous tissue proper, namely, the neurones and their processes. Neuroglia comprises three main types: astrocytes, oligodendroglia and microglia. The first two, sometimes referred to as macroglia, are derived from the middle layer of the neural tube, whilst microglia is of mesodermal origin. The three types of glia are morphologically distinguished, but require special techniques for their complete demonstration, only the nuclei being visible in such methods as haematoxylin and eosin. The ependymal cells lining the ventricles of the brain and the central canal of the spinal cord are also classified by some authorities under the heading of neuroglia.

See also Astrocytes; Oligodendroglia; Microglia.

Neurones

Nerve cells, varying considerably in shape and size, each consisting of a cell body containing a nucleus, and possessing cytoplasmic prolongations characteristically of two kinds: (1) a single axon or axis cylinder, often several feet in length, which conveys nervous impulses away from the cell, and (2) one or more shorter branching dendrites conveying impulses to the cell. Occurring in the cell body and passing through the processes are fine cytoplasmic fibrils often arranged in bundles, known as neurofibrils (q.v.). Chromidial or Nissl substance (q.v.) is also normally a prominent feature of the neurone, being found in the cytoplasm of the cell body and of the dendrites, but being absent from the axon. Pigment granules are sometimes present: melanin is found in certain cells, especially in the brain stem and in the locus coeruleus; lipofuscin is frequently present as a cytoplasmic inclusion and shows a gradual increase with advancing age. Demonstration of the specific components of the neurone is dealt with under the appropriate headings. The Bielschowsky group (q.v.) of techniques is of especial value for the neurone and its attendant processes.

Neurosecretory material (NSM)

A polypeptide hormonal secretion manufactured in the supra-optic and paraventricular nuclei of the hypothalamus and conveyed thence by means of the axons along the pituitary stalk for storage in the pars nervosa. The secretion includes the two hormones, oxytocin (responsible for smooth muscle contraction) and vaso-pressin (an antidiuretic and vasoconstrictor). Both of them were thought at one time to be products of the pars nervosa itself, rather than of the hypothalamus. A deficiency of neurosecretory material and consequently of these hormones, as a result of damage or malfunction of the posterior lobe of the pituitary or of the hypo-thalamus, may give rise to the condition known as diabetes insipidus. Neurosecretory material may be demonstrated histologically by chrome haematoxylin or by Gomori's aldehyde fuchsin.

Neutral fats

These are predominantly triglycerides of fatty acids, i.e. esters of the tri-hydroxy alcohol glycerol with, usually, palmitic, stearic (both saturated), or oleic (unsaturated) acids, or with mixtures of two or three of these. Stearodiolein, for example, an oleic-stearic-oleic triglyceride, is typical of human fat. Together with the ester waxes, esters of fatty acids with higher alcohols (e.g. cholesterol) they go to make up the class of simple lipids. Histologically they are sudanophil; they may be distinguished from the fatty acids by the Nile blue method (q.v.).

Neutral red

A basic dye of the azin subgroup of quinone-imine dyes. It is widely used as a red nuclear stain especially as a counterstain to blue- or violet-coloured elements, or to metallic impregnations. In the first group, for example, are the Gram methods for micro-organisms and Perls' Prussian blue reaction for iron; and the second group includes such techniques as von Kóssa for calcium, da Fano for Golgi apparatus, and many reticulin techniques. Staining may sometimes be enhanced by the addition of 1 per cent acetic acid. Neutral red is also used as an intra-vitam stain, often in conjunction with Janus green B. It forms the basis moreover, with light green, for Twort's neutral stain for parasites and bacteria.

Neutral red

Solubility at $20°C$ is 2.37 per cent in water and 2.0 per cent in alcohol.

Neutral stains

These are stain compounds formed by the interaction and precipitation of aqueous solutions of an acid and a basic dye, the precipitate being dried and dissolved in alcohol. Numerous combinations are possible: basic dyes such as methylene blue, basic fuchsin, neutral red, crystal violet, and methyl green; and acid dyes such as eosin, acid fuchsin, orange G, and light green, have all been employed. A mixture of the first example named in each selection (i.e. methylene blue and eosin) forms the basis for the valuable group of neutral stains, the Romanovsky group (q.v.).

Nicol prisms

An optical device consisting of two halves of a rhombohedral crystal of calcite (Iceland spar), cemented together with Canada balsam in such a way that a ray of light passing through it is split in two; one ray (ordinary ray) is totally reflected at the interface of the two halves, the other (extraordinary ray) passes through the prism as polarized light. In the polarizing microscope two such prisms are used, aligned in such a way that polarized light emerging from the one nearer the light source (polarizer) will pass freely through the second more remote one (analyser). If the latter is rotated through 90° the rays from the former will not pass through, the field being completely darkened; this is known as 'crossed Nicols'. If, however, a preparation containing birefringent material is introduced between the crossed Nicols, refraction of the polarized light occurs, causing the material to appear illuminated.

See Birefringence; Polaroid; Polarization of light.

Night blue

A basic dye of the phenyl methane group which has become popularized in recent years as an alternative to the Ziehl-Neelsen method for acid-fast bacilli; the organisms are stained blue followed by a red counterstain such as neutral red or safranin.

Night blue

Solubility at 20°C is 2.25 per cent in water and 2.35 per cent in alcohol.

Nile blue sulphate

A basic oxazin dye best known as a stain for lipid substances, introduced by Lorrain-Smith. Triglycerides or neutral fats are

coloured red or pink, and fatty acids, if liquid, coloured blue.
Phospholipids are usually stained blue, and cholesterol is unstained.

Nile blue sulphate

Nissl bodies (tigroid or chromidial substance)

Aggregations or granules of chromophil material found in the
cytoplasm of most nerve cells. It is invisible in the living cell, but is
seen by the electron microscope to consist of a protein framework of
parallel lamellae with numerous granules of RNA lying along and
between them. The significance of Nissl substance is as yet undeter-
mined, but it is thought to be concerned in the synthesis of cytoplasmic proteins. Its demonstration histologically may be effected in
tissue sections by the basic aniline dyes such as thionin, toluidin
blue, or neutral red, or by the pyronin component of the Unna-
Pappenheim stain (q.v.).

See also Neurones.

Nitric acid (HNO₃)

A colourless, highly corrosive liquid with a choking odour. It
should be stored in the dark to minimize generation of nitrogen
peroxide. Its main histological uses are: (1) as a decalcifying agent,
either as a simple aqueous dilution, usually 5 per cent, or stabilized
with urea, or in combination with chromic acid and alcohol as in
Perényi's fluid; (2) as a reagent for bile pigments (q.v.) in the Gmelin
reaction; and (3) in the preparation of the Millon reagent for
tyrosine.

Nitro dyes

A group of dyes characterized by the presence of the chromophoric NO_2 group. This chromophore is strongly acidic, hence the
dyes in this family are all acid dyes, the most commonly used being
trinitrophenol or picric acid. Other nitro dyes include aurantia
(q.v.) and Martius yellow.

Nuclear fast red

A basic dye, known often by its German name, Kernechtrot. It is
occasionally called for as a nuclear counterstain on frozen sections,
e.g. to Sudan black, behaving in a similar fashion to carmalum, in

that, as the term 'fast' implies, it is only removed with difficulty from aqueous-mounted sections. It should not be confused with the diazonium salt, variously known as Nuclear Fast Red Salt B, Kernechtrotsalz B, Fast Red Salt B, etc., which is dealt with under Diazo reaction (q.v.).

Nucleic acids
See Desoxyribonucleic acid; Ribonucleic acid.

Nucleolus
A small spheroidal body found within the cell nucleus, known sometimes as the plasmosome, and comprising a central core of ribonucleic acid (RNA) and a peripheral zone of desoxyribonucleic acid (DNA). They are said to be concerned with the synthesis of proteins. The plasmosome, or true nucleolus, should not be confused with the so-called karyosome, or false nucleolus, which is an agglomeration of chromatin.

Nucleoproteins
A group of conjugated proteins occurring in the cell nucleus, composed of nucleic acids in combination with basic proteins.

5-Nucleotidase
A substrate-specific phosphomonoesterase capable of splitting adenosine-5-phosphate (adenylic acid) at an optimum pH of 9.2. The enzyme has a fairly widespread distribution, notable sites being the tongue, liver, thyroid, and adrenal medulla.

Nucleotide
The fundamental unit of the complex double helix of the DNA molecule, comprising a phosphate, the sugar desoxyribose, and one of the four nitrogenous bases, adenine or guanine (purines), thymine or cytosine (pyrimidines).

Nucleus
A specialized part of the cell bounded by the nuclear membrane, and enclosing granules or strands of basophilic material (chromatin) and associated, usually spheroidal, nucleoli; all of these constituents lie in a colloidal protoplasm containing proteins and various salts. Most of the protein is bound to desoxyribonucleic acid (DNA) to form nucleoproteins, whose markedly acid reaction renders the nucleus readily demonstrable with basic dyes such as haematoxylin, the thiazins, neutral red, etc.
See also Chromosomes; Mitosis.

O

Oil red O

A weakly acid dye of the disazo group, used sometimes in preference to Sudans III and IV for the staining of fat because of its more intense red colour. It is usually employed in a solution of isopropanol, or in an acetone-alcohol mixture.

Oil red O

Oleic acid ($C_{17}H_{33}COOH$)

The commonest and most important of the unsaturated fatty acids, oleic acid is a constituent of human and other animal fats. It may occur as the free fatty acid or in its esterified form as a triglyceride in conjunction with the esters of stearic and/or palmitic acids. Such mixed triglycerides as stearodiolein (human fat) and oleopalmitobutyrin (butter) are readily isolated. Its most important histological significance is as a breakdown product of myelin, its properties as an unsaturated fatty acid being utilized in such methods as those of Marchi and Busch, which depend on its ability to reduce osmium tetroxide.

Oligodendroglia (Gk *oligos,* few + *dendron,* a tree)

A subdivision of neuroglial cells (oligodendrocytes), characterized by poorly developed processes, few in number, and not freely branched. Their nuclei are round or ovoid in contrast to those of microglia, which tend to be smaller and elongated. They are found abundantly in the white matter, often in rows between the myelinated fibre tracts and, less numerously in the grey matter, usually in the form of satellites to the neurones and blood vessels. Unlike the astrocytes their processes have no fibres and do not terminate in perivascular sucker feet or footplates. Their exact function is controversial, but they play a part in the enzyme balance of the myelin and tend to be much less numerous in myelin breakdown conditions, such as disseminated sclerosis and Schilder's encephalitis. Their demonstration is by no means easy: their processes degenerate rapidly after death and even when preserved may only be manifested by the metallic impregnation methods. The techniques are similar to those for showing microglia, but a more concentrated silver impregnating solution is sometimes helpful in such methods as Penfield, Hortega, and Weil-Davenport. Differentiation from microglia may be established also on morphological grounds.

See also Neuroglia; Microglia.

Orange G

An acid dye of the mono-azo group, widely used as a counterstain, either alone as in the Papanicolaou method, or in combination, e.g. in the Mallory connective tissue stains.

Orange G

Solubility at 20°C is 7.4 per cent in water and 0.35 per cent in alcohol.

Orcein

A weakly acid dye, originally derived from the lichen, *Lecanora tinctoria,* but nowadays the synthetic product is usually preferred. Its active ingredient is orcinol:

Orcinol

which, on oxidation and subsequent treatment with ammonia, is converted into orcein. Its main application in the histology laboratory is as a stain for elastic fibres, the solvent used being 1 per cent hydrochloric acid in 70 per cent alcohol.

Organelles

Specialized structural constituents of the cell, having some individual function, relating for example to metabolism, reproduction, or movement. They constitute the living material of the cell, in contrast to the inclusions, which are accumulations of non-living material, often of a temporary nature, e.g. glycogen and fat. The organelles include lysosomes, Golgi apparatus, mitochondria, etc., which are dealt with under the appropriate headings.

Osmium tetroxide (OsO_4)

A pale yellow crystalline solid with an acrid odour, loosely referred to as osmic acid. It should be treated with extreme caution as its vapour is highly injurious to the eyes, respiratory tract and skin. It should, moreover, be used sparingly as it is extremely costly; it is supplied in sealed ampoules, either 1.0 g or 0.1 g of the solid, or in aqueous solutions. It is a strong oxidant but is readily reduced by heat, light, or by organic or inorganic contaminants. Reduction may, however, be inhibited by the addition of a small quantity of mercuric chloride to the stock solution. The two important uses it has in histology are: (1) as a fixative, in which respect its preservative powers are excellent but its penetrant qualities are very poor so that small tissue blocks are essential (with these qualities it is finding current favour in electron microscopy); and (2) in the demonstration of lipids, which are both fixed and blackened, the tetroxide being reduced to a black oxide or hydroxide ($OsO_2 . 2H_2O$ or $Os(OH)_4$). This reaction is utilized in methods for the demonstration of degenerate myelin (e.g. Marchi) and of Golgi apparatus (e.g. Kolatchev). The vapour of osmium tetroxide, rather than the solution, is sometimes employed for the fixation of smears or small fragments of tissue and is called for in Cramer's method for the demonstration of adrenalin.

Osmosis

The phenomenon in which water or some other solvent passes through a semipermeable membrane from a weaker (hypotonic) to a stronger (hypertonic) solution until both solutions are of equal strength (isotonic). Histologically, osmosis is of especial importance in the action of fixing agents on the cell protoplasm.

Ovaries

The paired almond-shaped generative organs of the female, homologous with the male testes. They are concerned with the production of ova, each of which is invested with an epithelial sheath, the whole constituting a Graafian follicle. In the mature non-pregnant female one such follicle matures and ruptures through the ovarian surface at intervals of about 28 days, thus liberating an ovum. This process of ovulation leaves behind a scar on the surface of the ovary which becomes progressively more pitted. At the site of the rupture a small yellow endocrine body is formed, the corpus luteum, which is responsible for the secretion of the sex hormone, progesterone.

Oxalic acid (COOH.COOH)

A colourless crystalline poisonous compound, whose main uses in histology are: (1) as an integral part of the Mallory bleach (q.v.) following potassium permanganate; and (2) in the Weigert-Pal myelin techniques as a constituent, with potassium sulphite, of Pal's solution, which is used following differentiation in potassium permanganate to eliminate the brown colouration of the manganous compounds.

Oxazin dyes

One of the subdivisions of the quinone-imine group of dyes, characterized by the presence of the oxazin chromophoric group:

It includes such valuable nuclear stains as gallocyanin, celestin blue and cresyl violet, and also Nile blue sulphate.

Oxazones

A group of dyes derived from the oxazins (q.v.) by acid hydrolysis. The reaction is used histologically in the Nile blue technique for the differentiation of neutral fats from fatty acids. The red oxazone dye thus obtained is fat-soluble, the Nile blue itself being fat-insoluble but combining readily with free fatty acids to form a blue compound. A given globule, therefore, composed entirely of neutral fat will stain red and if composed of fatty acid will stain blue; mixtures of the two will exhibit a purplish colour varying in shade in proportion to the types of fat in the mixture. The efficacy of the staining solution may be tested by shaking up a few drops with xylene, the oxazone content being confirmed by the presence of a pink or red supernatant fluid.

Oxidation

A chemical process whereby a substance either (1) combines with oxygen, or (2) oxygen or some other electro-negative element is added to it, or (3) hydrogen or some other electro-positive element is removed from it. Oxidation procedures play a large part in histology, notably in the preparation of stains, e.g. haematoxylin, methylene blue, and the leuco-compounds such as leuco-fuchsin (Schiff's reagent) and leuco-patent blue; as a prelude to the demonstration of certain tissue elements, e.g. chromaffin and a number of enzymes and pigments; and as a preliminary to the visualization of argyrophil tissues such as reticulin and neurofibrils in metallic impregnations.

Oxidative enzymes

One of the main subdivisions of enzymes, including the oxidases, peroxidases, dehydrogenases, diaphorases, and tyrosinases. This field of enzyme histochemistry, particularly in respect of the dehydrogenases and diaphorases, has of recent years been expanded immeasurably by the introduction of substituted tetrazolium salts. The typical reaction is dependent upon the transfer of hydrogen from the enzyme-substrate combination and the consequent reduction of the colourless tetrazolium to the red-coloured formazan:

See also Cytochrome oxidase; Peroxidases; Tyrosinase; Dehydrogenases; Diaphorases.

P

Pancreas

A pinkish-white racemose gland lying in the retroperitoneum and intimately connected with the alimentary tract. It has a dual function being both exocrine, in that digestive juices, notably lipolytic and proteolytic enzymes are discharged into the duodenum, and endocrine, in that the islets of Langerhans (q.v.) are responsible for the secretion and discharge into the blood stream of insulin and other products such as glucagon and gastrin.

Paneth cells

Granular acidophilic epithelial cells usually found in groups, at the base of the crypts of Lieberkühn in the small intestine.
They are known to contain small amounts of zinc and their function may well represent a stage in the development of enzymes. They may be demonstrated by dyes of the eosin group, notably phloxine, as in the Lendrum's technique, using tartrazine as a differentiator.

Papanicolaou, George (1883–1962)

An American cytologist of Greek birth, he was first engaged on hormonal studies of vaginal smears from both animals and humans. During this work he noted the presence of cancer cells in smears and, recognizing the possibilities implicit in this observation, abandoned the purely endocrine aspect of his studies and concentrated thenceforth on the examination and classification of malignant cells from various sites. Despite the initial antagonism of pathologists and clinicians, his work has been fully vindicated and has proved of inestimable value, not only to medicine but to the community as a

whole. The ease with which large sections of the public may be
screened for the detection of early cancer, e.g. of cervix or lung is the
direct result of Papanicolaou's researches.
See also Exfoliative cytology.

Paraffin wax
See Waxes.

Paraldehyde (CH₃CHO)₃

A colourless hypnotic fluid, with an aromatic smell. It is used in
the preparation of Gomori's aldehyde fuchsin for the demonstration
of elastic fibres, mucins, and, perhaps more important, the β cells of
the pancreatic islets.

Pararosanilin

A constituent, together with one or more of its methylated
derivatives, of basic fuchsin (q.v.). Pararosanilin is triamino-triphenyl-
methane chloride.

Pararosanilin

Parathyroid glands

Small yellowish-brown bodies, usually four, occasionally five or
more, intimately connected with the posterior part of the thyroid
(q.v.). Their function is closely associated with calcium balance.

PAS (periodic acid-Schiff)

The most important and widely used of the oxidation-leucofuchsin
methods. It was initiated by McManus in 1946 for the purpose of
mucin demonstration (although Hotchkiss's work antedated this
publication, and moreover related to polysaccharides in general,
rather than to mucin in particular). The reaction is dependent on the
conversion by oxidation of 1:2-glycol groupings to aldehydes and
the subsequent formation of a reddish compound similar to, but not
identical with, basic fuchsin. Among the more important PAS
positive substances encountered histologically are the following:
epithelial mucins, glycogen, kidney basement membranes, basophil
cells of the pituitary, some lipofuscins and compound lipids, clubs in
actinomyces.

Patent blue V

An acid dye of the phenylmethane group, usually the calcium salt of:

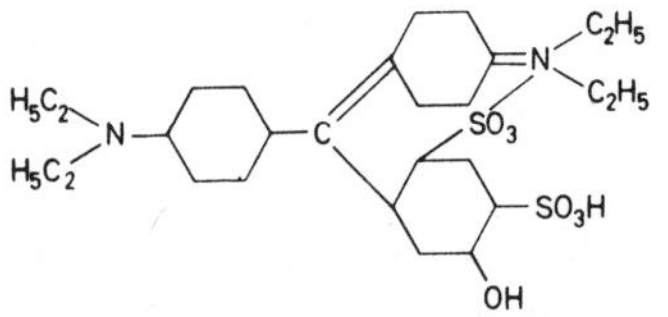

Patent blue V

Its most important application in histology is for the demonstration of haemoglobin peroxidase, the principal reagent being the leuco-form of the dye (*see* Leuco-dyes):

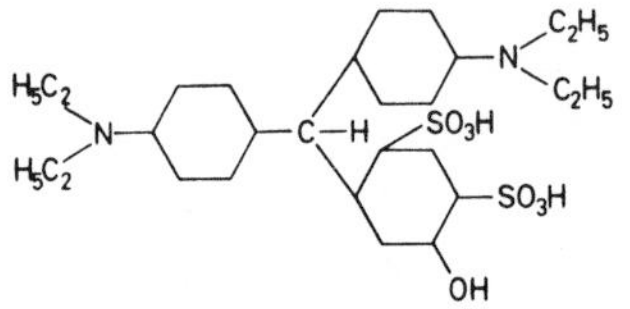

Leuco patent blue

This is prepared by boiling an aqueous solution of the dye with powdered zinc and acetic acid, the hydrogen thus liberated serving to break the chromophoric quinoid linkage and render the solution colourless. The colour is restored at the sites of peroxidase activity by the addition to the solution of hydrogen peroxide.

Perényi's fluid

A decalcifying solution with a rather slow, gentle action, containing chromic and nitric acids, and alcohol. It is ideally suited to the decalcification of bone marrow and other tissues containing small deposits of calcium.

Periodic acid ($HIO_4.2H_2O$)

A crystalline hygroscopic compound, soluble in water or alcohol, weakly acidic, easily reducible, and with important oxidant powers which are utilized in some Schiff techniques (q.v.) in which carbohydrates are oxidized to form aldehydes.

Perls, Max (1843–1881)

A German pathologist whose name (often mis-spelt as Perl) is associated with the Prussian blue reaction for haemosiderin (q.v.).

Peroxidase

A group of oxidative enzymes that catalyse the transfer of oxygen from hydrogen peroxide or from organic peroxides. They occur in granular leucocytes and erythrocytes and probably in the breast and thyroid; and in plant tissues as verdoperoxidase in seedlings and root vegetables, especially horseradish. Several methods have been used for their demonstration, notably those using benzidine, alpha-naphthol, or various leuco-dyes. Of these, the benzidine method, though effective, has fallen into disrepute owing to its carcinogenic nature, and the method of choice would appear to be the Lison-Dunn leuco-patent blue method.

PFAS (performic acid-Schiff)

A modification, together with the PAAS (Peracetic acid-Schiff), of the orthodox PAS method (q.v.) for the demonstration of ethylenic groups, which are present in unsaturated fatty acids, such as oleic, linoleic, linolenic, and arachidonic, all of which are probable constituents of the phospholipids, and some of them of the cerebrosides. The PFAS method is also of value in the manifestation of disulphide (-S-S-) and sulphydryl (-SH) groups in such organic compounds as cystine (SS) and cysteine and methionine (SH). These sulphur-containing amino acids occur widely in such tissues as skin (keratin), pancreatic beta cells (insulin), pituitary alpha cells (LTH, luteotrophin), hypothalamus (neurosecretory material – NSM), etc.

Phagocytosis

The ingestion by certain macrophage-type cells of the reticulo-endothelial system or by leucocytes, of foreign particles, micro-organisms, spermatozoa, etc. The phenomenon is utilized histologic-ally in the study of the reticuloendothelial system by the injection of certain vital dyes, such as trypan blue, particles of which are engulfed by the phagocytes. Subsequent processing and sectioning of such tissues reveals the nature and distribution of these cells.

Phenol (C_6H_5OH)

A colourless crystalline solid, turning pink on exposure to air; it is poisonous and caustic. Histologically its main uses are as an accentua-tor, e.g. in carbol fuchsin and carbol thionin; as a preservative in staining and other reagent solutions; and for the softening of hard tissues prior to paraffin embedding.

Phenyl methane dyes

A very important group of dyes, based on a central carbon atom, with two or three of the four attached hydrogen atoms, characteristic of methane, being replaced by phenyl groups:

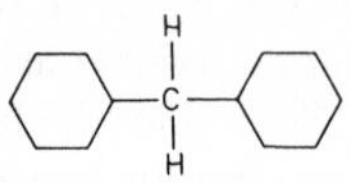

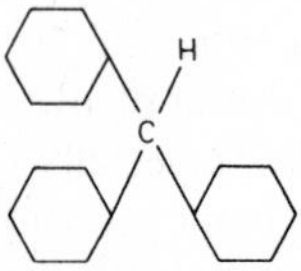

Diphenyl methane   *Triphenyl methane*

A rearrangement of each of these molecules takes place on oxidation, a residual hydrogen atom being removed and a powerful chromophoric compound being thus formed:

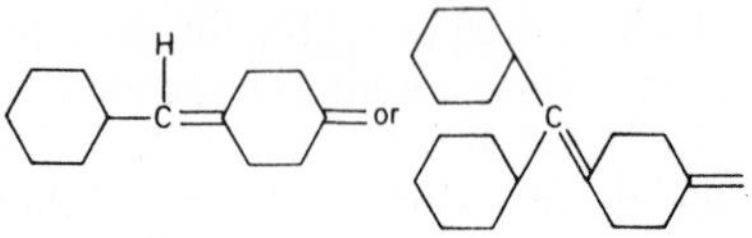

The group includes such widely-used dyes as basic and acid fuchsins, methyl and crystal violets, light green, patent blue, aniline blue and Victoria blue, and the notable fluorochrome, auramine.

Phloxine

A member of the fluorescein sub-group of xanthene dyes. The eosins, erythrosins and rose bengals complete the group. It may replace eosin as a red counterstain, but is of especial value in the demonstration of Paneth cell granules and certain inclusion bodies, e.g. in Lendrum's phloxine-tartrazine method, the staining solution used being 0.5 per cent phloxine in 0.5 per cent calcium chloride.

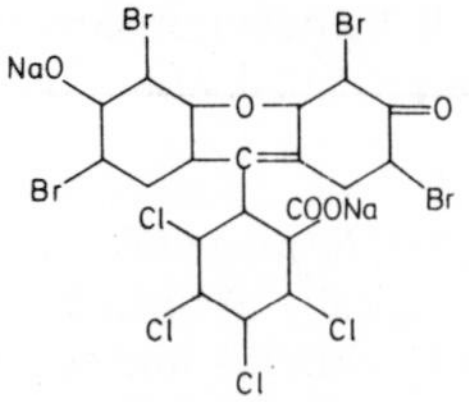

Phloxine

Solubility at $20°C$ is 39.25 per cent in water, 7.0 per cent in alcohol, and 2.4 per cent in cellosolve.

Phosphamidase

A substrate-specific phosphomonoesterase capable of splitting p-chloroanilidophosphoric acid at a pH of 5.6. It occurs in the grey matter of the nervous system, especially of the cerebellum, and in malignant epithelial cells.

Phosphatides (*Synonym:* Phospholipids)
    See Phospholipids.

Phosphine 3R
    A basic dye of the acridine subgroup of the xanthenes, it is of value in the examination of lipids by fluorescence microscopy. It is a derivative of chrysanilin, probably a mixture of nitrates.

Phosphine 3R

    A secondary silvery-white fluorescence is exhibited by simple and compound lipids, but not by derived lipids, namely fatty acids and cholesterol.

Phospholipids
    Known variously as phospholipins and phosphatides, these are physiologically the most important of the body lipids. They are essential constituents of every living cell, but exist largely in 'masked' form, often in conjunction with other lipid and non-lipid elements. This intimate association may be broken, sometimes pathologically (by bacterial or chemical intoxications), or by technical processes such as chemical treatment, heat, etc. Thus red blood corpuscles, while not reacting with Sudan black B in frozen sections, are readily demonstrable in paraffin sections by the same stain. The lecithins consist of glycerol, fatty acids, phosphoric acid, and the nitrogenous base choline; the cephalins are found in association with lecithins, but differ from them in the possession of ethanolamine instead of choline as the basic nitrogen compound. The third group, the sphingomyelins, although possessing a phosphoric acid group have more in common with the cerebrosides (q.v.) and in some modern classifications are indeed listed with them. Both the sphingomyelins and the cerebrosides contain a sphingosine molecule representing the nitrogenous fraction, and replacing glycerol. Choline, moreover, is present in the sphingomyelins. Identification of individual phospholipids poses numerous problems, but differential extraction techniques, often in association with staining methods such as

Baker's acid haematein and McManus Sudan black B, may offer valuable information.

Phosphomonoesterases

One of the main subdivisions of hydrolytic enzymes, the two most important of which are alkaline phosphatase (phosphomono-esterase I) and acid phosphatase (phosphomonoesterase II). Each of these groups in turn may be further broken down into non-specific and specific varieties. The non-specific phosphatases will hydrolyse a variety of orthophosphate esters, the alkaline phosphatases operating best at pH 9.0 or over, the acid phosphatases at about pH 5.0.

See also Alkaline phosphatase; 5-Nucleotidase; Aldolase; Adenosine triphosphatase; Acid phosphatase; Phosphamidase; Glucose-6-phosphatase.

Picric acid $(C_6H_2(NO_2)_3OH)$

A yellow acid dye, trinitrophenol, of the nitro group, sometimes used alone as a counterstain, more often with other acid dyes such as acid fuchsin or orange G. It stains muscle and erythrocytes bright yellow. It also figures in some methods as a differentiator, notably in Schmorl's picrothionin method for bone canaliculi, in Altmann's aniline-acid fuchsin for mitochondria, and as an alternative to iron alum following Heidenhain's haematoxylin for muscle striations, etc. Its fixative properties are considerable; it is a powerful protein precipitant and is employed in Bouin's fluid and its variants as a general fixative, and especially as a preservative for glycogen. Moreover it has some value as a mordant, especially for acid dyes, where it may be used as a separate solution or incorporated in the fixative.

Picric acid

Picric acid is explosive when heated or on detonation, and for safety should be stored and transported moistened with water.

Pigments

In histology, those substances which are rendered visible by virtue of their own colour, which may be intensified or otherwise altered by chemical means, visualization being thus facilitated. They are usually classified as (1) artefact pigments, which may occur as products of fixation, e.g. acid formaldehyde haematin (q.v.); (2) endogenous pigments, which are engendered within the organism by metabolic processes – these include the blood pigments (q.v.), melanin and the lipofuscins; and (3) exogenous pigments, which are introduced from without, either as occupational or environmental hazards, from dietary sources, or even, in the case of tattoo pigments, by design!

Pineal body

A small, grey conical body attached by the pineal stalk to the roof of the third ventricle of the brain. It is probably the vestige of the third eye, representing a functioning organ in reptiles and amphibia that are now extinct. There is some evidence to suggest that an association exists between the pineal and male sexual development, but the nature and significance of this association is still obscure.

Pituitary

This small rounded endocrine gland, called sometimes the hypophysis cerebri, lies at the base of the brain in a small cavity of the sphenoid bone. It is attached to the brain by a slender stalk (the pars tuberalis) and consists of two main lobes, the anterior and posterior lobes, separated by an intermediate zone (pars intermedia). The anterior lobe (pars anterior) is made up of three main types of cell, the acidophil or alpha cells, the basophil or beta cells, and the chromophobe cells. The acidophils and basophils are together responsible for the secretion of a wide range of hormones, although the separate functions of each type is by no means agreed. The chromophobes on the other hand are thought to be non-secretory. The posterior lobe (pars nervosa) consists, as the name implies, of nervous tissue, the main cells being the pituicytes, which are essentially modified neuroglial cells. The most important function of the pars nervosa is the storage of two hormones: vasopressin, with antidiuretic and vasoconstrictor properties; and oxytocin, which causes contraction of the smooth muscle. These two hormones are constituents of neurosecretory material (NSM), manufactured in the hypothalamus and conveyed through the pituitary stalk to the pars nervosa of the pituitary. The pars intermedia is said to be responsible, certainly in reptiles, amphibians and some of the lower mammals, for the elaboration of a specific hormone causing expansion of melanocytes and consequent darkening of the skin. Methods used for the demonstration of the cells of the pituitary include those of the trichrome group, especially the Crooke-Russell modification of Mallory's connective tissue stain (AFAB), and the PAS method, the acidophil cells being counterstained with orange G.

See also Acidophil; Basophil.

111

Placenta

The afterbirth, a thick fleshy disc about 7 in in diameter which is attached during pregnancy to the uterine wall of the mother and connected to the foetus by the umbilical cord. It comprises a complex system of vascular processes, its primary function being to permit diffusion of dissolved substances from the foetal to the maternal blood and vice versa. This diffusion is controlled by means of a cellular membrane known as the placental barrier. The placenta also possesses certain endocrine properties and is responsible for the secretion of oestrogen and other hormones and enzymes.

Plasma cells

A special type of connective tissue cell, found commonly in haemopoietic tissues and in serous membranes. Their occurrence in normal loose connective tissue is comparatively rare, but there is marked proliferation in chronic inflammatory lesions. The appearance of a plasma cell is distinctive: the cell is rounded with a spherical, eccentrically-placed nucleus having a characteristic chromatin pattern aggregated into coarse peripheral clumps, often likened to a clock face or cart wheel. The cytoplasm is strongly basophil and homogeneous with a high RNA content. Their demonstration in tissue sections may be carried out by the Unna-Pappenheim pyronin and methyl green method or one of its modifications, e.g. Trevan and Sharrock.

Plasmal reaction

A histochemical technique for the demonstration of plasmalogens or acetal phosphatides which differ from true phospholipids, such as lecithin and cephalin, in that two of the hydroxyl groups of the tri-hydroxy alcohol glycerol are bound by acetal linkage to one fatty aldehyde; the third hydroxyl group is esterified by a phosphoric radical which is itself tied to the nitrogenous base.

$$
\begin{array}{l}
CH_2O \\
\quad\quad\ \ \searrow CH.R \text{ (fatty acid)} \\
CHO \nearrow \\
CH_2O - P \!=\! O \\
\quad\quad\quad\quad\ \ \ \text{OH} \\
\quad\quad\quad\quad O - CH_2 \\
\quad\quad\quad\quad\quad\quad | \\
\quad\quad\quad\quad\quad\quad CH_2 \ \text{(ethanolamine)} \\
\quad\quad\quad\quad\quad\quad | \\
\quad\quad\quad\quad\quad\quad NH_2
\end{array}
$$

The method consists of treating fresh unfixed frozen sections or smears with a dilute (1 per cent) solution of mercuric chloride, the aldehydes thereby being released and readily demonstrable by Schiff's reagent.

Polaroid

A material used in polariscopy as a substitute for the Nicol prism system, in the form of celluloid- or glass-covered discs. They consist of a suspension of ultramicroscopic crystals of quinine iodosulphate (herapathite, $4C_{20}H_{24}O_2N_2.3H_2SO_4.2HI.2I_2.6H_2O$) in nitrocellulose. Herapathite crystals are themselves not only birefringent but have the property of transmitting only the extraordinary rays, the ordinary rays being absorbed. The crystals are orientated in such a fashion that their optical paths are parallel. Mounted between glass or celluloid sheeting they act as a single crystal. As in the case of Nicol prisms, two such discs are necessary, one acting as polarizer, the other as analyser.

See also Nicol prisms; Birefringence; Herapathite.

Polarization of light

See Nicol prisms.

Polyethylene glycols ($C_{2n}H_{4n}O_{n-1}(OH)_2$)

The water-soluble or carbowaxes, used for tissue embedding, form a range of carbohydrates with varying physical properties, those with low molecular weights (from 200 to 700) being liquid, those with heavier molecules becoming progressively more solid (from 800 upwards). Esters of these compounds with fatty acids (e.g. stearic) are also employed. The cardinal virtue of the carbowaxes is their miscibility with water, so that the intermediate processes of dehydration and clearing are automatically eliminated and *ipso facto* the shrinkage and distortion that they engender. The carbowaxes are miscible with alcohol, xylene, the aromatic oils, and water, but not with benzene, ether, or paraffin wax. Moreover they are miscible with each other to give intermediate physical properties. The blocks obtained by these techniques are of a hard paraffin-like consistency and lend themselves readily to ribboning. Floating out the sections presents difficulties, in that they disintegrate in contact with water, and a 20 per cent solution of polyethylene glycol 900 and various detergents have been recommended. Blocks should be stored temporarily in a desiccator and for permanent storage invested with a thin layer of paraffin wax. The methods have been applied to the study of lipids and enzymes and also in the realm of dental histology.

Post-chroming

The treatment with a solution containing a chrome salt, usually potassium dichromate, of tissue or tissue sections following normal fixation. Various applications of this procedure are recommended,

113

primarily for mordanting effect, in techniques for the demonstration of mitochondria, of myelin and other lipids, of chromaffin substance, and in such routine staining methods as PTAH (q.v.) and the trichrome group.

Potassium dichromate ($K_2Cr_2O_7$)

A bright orange-red crystalline compound, soluble in water to about 12 per cent at room temperature. It is extensively used as a fixative, usually in combination with such reagents as mercuric chloride, formaldehyde and osmium tetroxide. Its behaviour is dependent on the pH at which it is employed: when strongly acid (below pH 4.5) it has an action similar to that of chromic acid and preserves chromosomes and the chromatin network, but mitochondria are destroyed. At a less acid pH, mitochondria are well fixed but at the expense of the nucleoproteins. Tissues should be thoroughly washed in running water before dehydration with alcohol. Apart from its uses as a primary fixative it has found favour in recent years as a secondary fixative following formaldehyde. Potassium dichromate possesses powerful mordanting properties, whether it is (1) incorporated in the fixative; (2) used as a separate solution following fixation of the tissue block; or (3) used as a solution for treatment of cut paraffin or frozen sections prior to staining. A further use, in conjunction with concentrated sulphuric acid, is for cleaning glassware. Extreme caution should be exercised in preparing or handling this mixture.

Potassium permanganate ($KMnO_4$)

A dark purple crystalline compound, it is a valuable oxidant, widely used in histology. It is an integral part of the 'Mallory bleach' (q.v. under Mallory, Frank), an oxidation sequence comprising iodine, sodium thiosulphate, potassium permanganate, and oxalic acid. The permanganate-oxalic acid sequence is also used as a differentiator in the Weigert-Pal techniques for myelin, and in order to bleach pigments such as melanin. Alone it is sometimes employed as an oxidant for haematoxylin solutions, e.g. Mallory's phosphotungstic acid—haematoxylin, and either alone or acidified as an oxidant prior to reticulin impregnations and in some oxidation-Schiff procedures.

Processing

A histological term, known in the vernacular as 'putting through'. It is sometimes taken to mean the entire process of preparation of the tissues prior to section cutting and staining, from fixation to embedding inclusive; some, however, regard it as denoting only the stages of dehydration, clearing, and impregnation.

Progressive staining
See Regressive staining.

Prophase
The initial stage of cell division or mitosis in which the chromatin becomes concentrated into a tangled mass of filaments, which resolve themselves into pairs of chromosomes. The centriole meanwhile has divided, each half moving to opposite poles of the cell and being joined by a number of delicate fibres known as the achromatic spindle (q.v.), along which the paired chromosomes become orientated.

Propylene glycol ($CH_3.CHOH.CH_2OH$)
A hygroscopic viscous fluid miscible with acetone, chloroform, and water and preferred by some authorities as a solvent for fat stains such as Sudan III and Sudan black, giving an intense colouration with minimal loss of fat.

Prostate
A gland constituting part of the male reproductive system. It surrounds the neck of the urinary bladder and is traversed by the urethra and the ejaculatory ducts. It secretes a thin opalescent liquid which forms a fluid medium for the transmission of spermatozoa; because of its alkaline reaction it neutralizes the effects of urinary remnants from the urethra and the strongly acid vaginal mucus.

Prussian blue $Fe_4(Fe(CN)_6)_3$
The common name for ferric ferrocyanide which is the histochemical end-product in Perls' reaction for the demonstration of iron pigment.

PTAH
A universally accepted abbreviation denoting Mallory's phosphotungstic acid—haematoxylin method. This technique has a very wide application in the histology laboratory, particularly as a stain for neuroglia, fibrin and muscle striations. It will also demonstrate such diverse structures as fibroglia, myofibrils, prickle borders of epithelial cells, blepharoplasts, mitochondria, and bile canaliculi.

Purines
Organic bases which, like the pyrimidines, are produced on acid hydrolysis of nucleic acids.

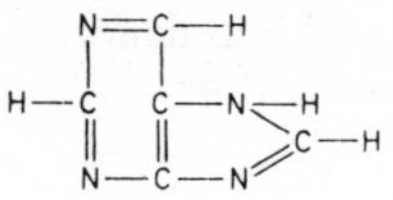

N≡C—H
H—C C—N—H
N—C—N C—H

Purine

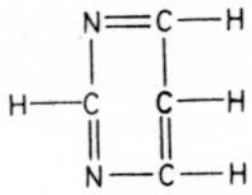

N≡C—H
H—C C—H
N—C—H

Pyrimidine

As yet no means seem to have been devised for their specific demonstration.

Purkinje, Johannes Evangelista (1787–1869)

A Bohemian physiologist and a notable pioneer in the realm of microtomy, being the first to cut tissue sections with a microtome instead of freehand, and also the first to use Canada balsam as a mountant. He gave his name to the large cerebellar neurones and also to certain atypical cardiac fibres. Moreover, he was probably the first to recognize the importance of fingerprints.

Purpurin

An acid dye of the anthraquinone group, which includes the popular stains for calcium notably alizarin (q.v.).

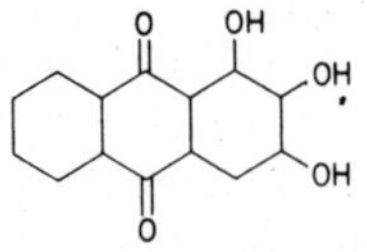

Purpurin

Solubility at 20°C is 0.7 per cent in alcohol.

Pyknosis

The dark-staining shrunken appearance of nuclei as a result of nuclear condensation following cell death. It is a term widely used in cytology and refers especially to the cornified superficial squamous cells of the vagina etc.

Pyridine ($C_5 H_5 N$)

An inflammable colourless liquid with a characteristic pungent smell. It is a powerful fat solvent and figures in lipid extraction techniques, notably in Baker's method for the demonstration of phospholipids (q.v.). It is also widely used in metallic methods, notably for CNS, in order to minimize background impregnation and scum formation and its attendant precipitation. It is highly toxic and is a skin irritant.

Pyrimidines

See Purines.

Pyronin

A basic dye of the xanthene group, its main application is in the Unna-Pappenheim method and its variants for plasma cells, bacteria, RNA, and DNA. It is extensively used for the demonstration of Nissl substance with its high RNA content.

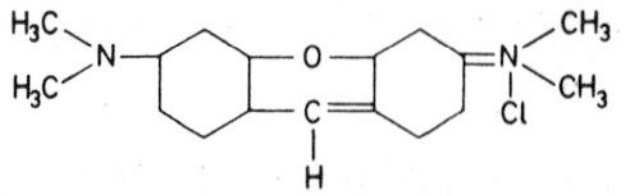

Pyronin Y (or G)

Solubility at 20°C is 9.0 per cent in water and 0.60 per cent in alcohol.

Q

Quenching

See Freeze drying.

Quinone ($C_6H_4O_2$)

An oxidizing agent derived from benzene and of great importance in dye chemistry for its chromophoric properties. The configuration known as the quinoid linkage occurs, sometimes modified, in several dye families known collectively as the quinone-imine dyes (q.v.).

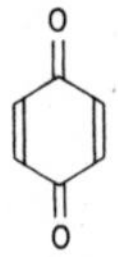

Quinoid linkage

Quinone-imine dyes

A large and very important family of dyes containing both the indamin (−N=) and quinoid chromophoric groups. These dyes may be subdivided into five subgroups, three of which are of considerable significance: the azins, the oxazins, and the thiazins. Each of these is dealt with under its appropriate heading.

R

Radioisotope

An isotope (q.v.) which has been rendered radioactive, usually by artificial means, and has the ability to decompose spontaneously, thus becoming radio-inactive. The introduction of such isotopes ('tracer elements') into the body by oral or parenteral means enables their ultimate distribution to be detected by a Geiger counter (q.v.) or by autoradiography (q.v.). Examples of such substances used in medical investigations are radio-iodine (I^{131}) for thyroid function, radio-calcium (Ca^{45}) in studies of calcium absorption, and radio-potassium (K^{42}) for the study of potassium exchange.

Regressive staining

This entails staining for a prolonged time, followed by the selective removal of the stain by a decolourizing fluid, the latter procedure being known as differentiation. This mode of staining, as distinct from progressive staining which requires periodical inspection of the preparation until the required intensity is achieved, is in general much more satisfactory in that it permits better control of the end result. Moreover, differentiation is an effective means of eliminating undesirable background colouration and of ensuring a cleaner, crisper picture. A limited number of stains do not, however, lend themselves to this treatment and must be employed progressively (for example, Mallory's phosphotungstic acid—haematoxylin). Others are essentially regressive stains, notably Heidenhain's iron alum haematoxylin; the controlled differentiation of this stain may allow the demonstration successively of such diverse elements as mitochondria, muscle striations, chromatin, and nucleoli. Nevertheless, the vast majority of stains, including most of the haematoxylin solutions, may be used in either fashion.

Resins

A generic term used to cover a wide range of substances, natural and synthetic, the natural resins being exudates of plants, the synthetic of similar nature but obtained by chemical means. They are, in contrast to the gums, insoluble in water. Resins may be used as constituents of mounting media, both for microscopy and museum specimens; as embedding substances, especially in the preparation of ultra-thin sections for the electron microscope; and, in the case of ion-exchange resins, for decalcification.

See also Acrylic resins; Decalcification; Epoxy resins; Mounting media.

Reticular fibres

These elements of connective tissue are often loosely referred to as 'reticulin' which perhaps more accurately should be confined to the constituent protein. A long-standing controversy still rages over their relationship with collagen fibres; although reticular fibres possess a strong argyrophilia and collagen fibres do not (thus indicating some fundamental but as yet hypothetical chemical difference), examination under the electron microscope shows no basic structural dissimilarity. Their function is that of a delicate supporting framework for cells, capillaries, glandular secretory units, and as a boundary between connective and other types of tissues.

As indicated above, their demonstration is best effected by impregnation with an ammoniacal silver solution in such techniques as Gomori, Gordon and Sweet, Foot, etc. They may also be stained by the trichrome methods and by PAS.

Reticulin

See Reticular fibres.

Rhodamines

A subgroup of the xanthene family of dyes, similar to the pyronins, but possessing a third benzene ring replacing the attached hydrogen atom:

Rhodamines

Their main histological use is in fluorescence microscopy.

Ribonucleic acid (RNA)

One of the two vital nucleic acids, the other being desoxyribonucleic acid (DNA). RNA was at one time thought to be confined to plant tissues, notably yeast, but is now established as an essential constituent of the nucleolus and cytoplasm of all animal cells. Its chemical composition resembles that of DNA (q.v.), but differs from it in the nature of the pentose sugar and of one of the pyrimidine bases, RNA being characterized by uracil instead of DNA's thymine. Ribonucleic acid may be demonstrated histologically by the Unna-Pappenheim method (q.v.) or by fluorescence techniques using acridine orange; RNA exhibits a red and DNA a green fluorescence.

Ringing media

These are cements which are applied to the edge of the coverslip in order to prevent evaporation or bubble formation in the mounting medium. They are of special value in the case of aqueous mountants. A wide variety of substances has been used including paraffin wax, gold size, asphalt varnish, colophonium wax, cellulose paint, and plastic cements.

119

Ripening

A widely-used colloquial term for the maturation or oxidation of certain dye solutions, notably of haematoxylin (q.v.). The process occurs spontaneously but may be accelerated by the addition of such oxidants as sodium iodate, potassium permanganate, or mercuric oxide. Such artificial ripening produces optimum staining power in a short time but, unless controlled carefully, carries with it the danger of over-oxidation. The term 'ripening' is often extended to include the polychroming of methylene blue which again is an oxidative process, the stain which is a tetramethyl thionin being converted in part to the dimethyl and trimethyl thionins (Azure A and Azure B).

See Methylene blue; Haematoxylin.

Romanovsky, Dmitri Leonidovitch (1861–1921)

A Russian physician, and the originator (in 1891) of a technique utilizing a mixture of aqueous solutions of eosin and methylene blue for the purpose of staining blood films, with particular reference to malarial parasites. Innumerable modifications were subsequently devised including the precipitation and resolution of the compound dye in alcohol, and the artificial oxidation or 'polychroming' of the methylene blue. Such well-known variants as Jenner (1899), Leishman (1901), and Wright (1902) were based directly upon the parent method, whilst Giemsa, Maximow, and others used oxidation products of methylene blue as a starting point for their variants. The entire range of methods is sometimes known as the Romanovsky group.

Rosanilin

A phenyl methane dye and commonly a constituent of basic fuchsin, it is monomethyl fuchsin:

Rosanilin

Solubility at $20°C$ is 0.39 per cent in water and 8.16 per cent in alcohol.

Rose Bengal

An acid dye of the xanthene group, and of less importance than

the other members, the eosins, erythrosins, and phloxines. It is
distinguished from these by the presence of chlorine and iodine
atoms in the molecule.

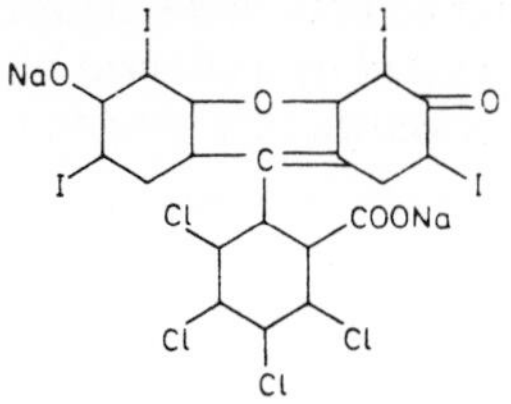

Rose bengal

Solubility at 20°C is 36 per cent in water and 7.5 per cent in
alcohol.

S

Saffron

A natural dye extracted from a species of crocus, whose properties have been recognized for several thousand years. Histologically
it is of interest as probably the first recorded instance of a dye
substance being employed for microbiological purposes, since it was
used by Leeuwenhoek, 'the father of the microscope', for staining
bovine muscle.

Safranins

A subdivision of the azin dyes, one of the nitrogen atoms of the
chromophore being pentavalent and having an attached benzene
ring. Safranin is a powerful basic red dye and is often used as a
nuclear counterstain, e.g. in Gram's methods for micro-organisms.

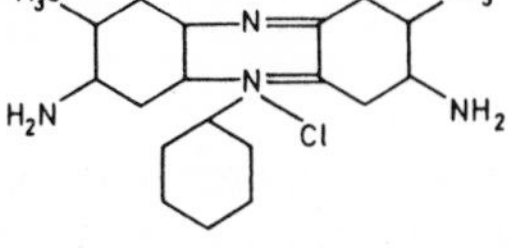

Safranin O

Solubility at 20°C is 6.25 per cent in water and 2.0 per cent in
alcohol.

Salivary glands

Three large paired glands, parotid, submaxillary and sublingual,
and numerous small accessory glands opening on to the mucous
membranes of the cheeks, tongue, floor of mouth and palate, and
discharging their secretions (saliva) by means of salivary ducts into

the oral cavity. The glands are composed of groups of secretory cells, mucous and serous, known as alveoli, which may be of three types, wholly mucous, wholly serous, or mixed mucous and serous. This last type of mixed alveolus is found only in the submaxillary and sublingual glands and is characterized by a crescent of serous cells capping a group of mucous cells known as a crescent of Giannuzzi or demilune of Heidenhain.

Scarlet red
See Sudan IV.

Scharlach R
See Sudan IV.

Schaudinn's fluid
A cytological fixative containing mercuric chloride, alcohol, and usually a trace of acetic acid. It is unsuitable for use with blocks of tissue because of the considerable shrinkage and distortion, its main applications being in cytology and protozoology for the fixation of smear preparations. The mercury content necessitates treatment of the fixed smears with iodized alcohol.

Schiff, Hugo (1834–1915)
A German biochemist whose reagent for aldehydes is based on the formation of a leucofuchsin, obtained by the decolourization of basic fuchsin by sulphurous acid. The quinoid structure is thus broken, but is restored in the presence of aldehydes. The reagent has a growing application in widely divergent fields of histochemistry: (1) in the Feulgen reaction (q.v.) for chromatin (or more specifically DNA), devised in 1924; (2) in the periodic acid-Schiff (PAS) reaction (q.v.); (3) in modifications of this such as the performic acid-Schiff (PFAS) and peracetic acid-Schiff (PAAS) reactions (q.v.); and (4) in the plasmal reaction (q.v.).
See also Leuco dyes.

Schmorl, Christian Georg (1861–1932)
A Dresden pathologist, who made many valuable contributions in the field of histological theory and practice. His standard work *Histopathological Research Methods* ran into 11 editions from 1897 to 1934 and included many of his own techniques, some of which remain firmly established in the current repertoire. The best known are his techniques for bone canaliculi using thionin or picrothionin, and his ferric chloride-potassium ferricyanide mixture for reducing substances such as lipofuscin and melanin. This reagent, although usually attributed to Schmorl, was in fact devised some years earlier (1909) by Golodetz and Unna.

Secondary fixation

The treatment of tissues after initial fixation in formalin with some other fixing solution, usually containing mercuric chloride and/or potassium dichromate, which is designed to improve or facilitate the demonstration of general or specific tissue elements.

Serial sections

A term used to denote a sequence of sections, either complete and uninterrupted, or at predetermined regular intervals, in order to examine a small lesion or other tract of tissue in considerable detail. Such study may be carried out readily with paraffin material in that ribbons are easily produced, and a strict numerical sequence controlled. In the absence of suitable paraffin material, other methods, such as celloidin, LVN, or frozen sections, are sometimes called for, but pose serious problems in that sections are of necessity obtained singly; hence great care must be taken to ensure that no disruption of the sequence occurs. Such devices as the adhesion of sections to a celloidin-covered glass plate or photo-film, the interleaving of sections between numbered tissue papers, or direct adhesion to numbered albuminized slides can sometimes minimize the difficulties.

Sex chromatin

An aggregation of chromatin representing the XX pair of chromosomes which may be seen at the periphery of interphase nuclei of female cells. This condensation of chromatin is known as the Barr body, and may readily be seen in smear preparations (e.g. of buccal or vaginal mucosa in 40 to 60 per cent of female cells). In the chromosomal male the normal percentage is below 15 per cent. The prominence of the Barr body may be explained by the fact that the X chromosome is very much larger than the Y; hence in female cells the XX pair is more readily visible than the XY. Special methods include cresyl fast violet acetate and Guard's method using Biebrich scarlet and fast green FCF. In stained blood films the polymorphonuclear neutrophils manifest the Barr body in the form of a drumstick attached by a delicate thread to the lobulated nucleus.

Skin

The integument or outer covering of the body comprising two layers: an outer epidermis and an inner corium or dermis, together with the skin appendages. The epidermis consists of stratified squamous epithelium, composed of up to five layers; (1) the deepest, the germinal layer (stratum germinativum) abutting on the dermis, responsible for the manufacture of new cells and of the pigment melanin. These new cells are promoted to the next layer, (2) the

123

prickle-cell layer (stratum spinosum), several cells deep, which in turn merges into (3) the stratum granulosum, so called because of the haematoxyphil granules of keratohyalin present in the cell cytoplasm. Superficial to this are two layers of dead cells: (4) the stratum lucidum, a clear eosinophil layer, and finally (5) the horny layer (stratum corneum), composed of keratinized cells that ultimately desquamate from the surface. All five layers are present only in those areas subjected to heavy wear and tear, namely the palms of the hands and soles of the feet. The dermis is formed of two poorly demarcated layers of connective tissue, the papillary layer interdigitating with the epidermis, and the thicker reticular layer deep to it, each with a plentiful supply of blood vessels. The skin appendages include sweat glands, sebaceous glands, hair follicles and nails. The functions of the skin are multiple and diverse: (1) it is protective, insofar as it is a barrier to micro-organisms, is almost waterproof, and, by virtue of the melanin in the germinal layer is a safeguard against excessive sunlight; (2) sensory, receiving various stimuli from outside and transmitting them to the brain; (3) excretory, since it expels by means of sweat, water and other waste products contained therein; and (4) thermostatic, as it facilitates heat loss by radiation, or conversely can insulate against cold.

Sodium hydrosulphite ($Na_2S_2O_4$)

A white crystalline powder, known also, and more correctly, as sodium dithionite. It is used in histology as an alternative to alcohol in the Kaiserling methods and their variants, for the restoration of colour in museum specimens.

Solochrome cyanin

A dye of the phenyl methane group soluble in alcohol or water, and increasingly popular as a relatively rapid and simple stain for the demonstration of myelin, iron alum acting as both mordant and differentiator. It may also be employed for the demonstration of osteoid tissue in bone, for the visualization of aluminium in tissues, or simply, in phosphoric acid solution, as a nuclear stain.

Solochrome cyanin

Solubility at 20°C is 7.2 per cent in water and 5.1 per cent in alcohol.

Solochrome prune

A dye in current favour as an alternative to celestine blue or gallocyanin for the staining of chromatin.

The stain is prepared in the form of its iron lake by boiling with ferric ammonium alum.

Spalteholz

The name given to a technique whereby gross specimens are rendered transparent. The method normally follows the injection of opaque-coloured media into a vascular or other intraluminal system. It involves fixation, scrupulous dehydration in graded alcohols, clearing in benzene, and treatment with benzyl benzoate, to which methyl salicylate (oil of wintergreen) is later added, the specimen being mounted in a mixture of the two.

See also Injection methods.

Sphingolipids

A generic name given to the sphingosine-containing compound lipids which is gaining currency and is recommended by such an eminent authority as Lison. Included in the group are the sphingo-myelins and the cerebrosides (q.v.), namely kerasin, phrenosin and nervon. The sphingosine base is as follows:

$$CH_3(CH_2)_{12}HC = CH.CHOH.CH(NH_2)CH_2OH$$

As with the phospholipids, they may be recognized by differential extraction methods in conjunction with staining and histo-chemical manifestation.

Spinal cord

That part of the central nervous system extending downwards from the brain stem and ending in the filum terminale in the region of the coccyx, the whole being enclosed within the vertebral column. The cord is divided into four regions; cervical, thoracic, lumbar and sacral. Each of these possesses its own distinctive cross section, in respect of size, shape, proportion of white matter to grey, etc. Peripherally, the spinal cord consists of white matter, composed of bundles of myelinated nerve fibres longitudinally arranged, enclosing a central core of grey matter. This is roughly H-shaped, the cross bar being known as the commissure, and the poles of the lateral bars as the left and right anterior and posterior horns. The characteristic cells of the grey matter are large neurones (q.v.).

Spirochaetes

The organisms in this group most commonly encountered in

histology are *Trepenema pallidum* and *Leptospira icterohaemorrhagica,* the causative organisms of syphilis and Weil's disease respectively. Demonstration may be effected either by block impregnation in silver nitrate and reduction in pyrogallol or similar reducer (Levaditi and modifications), or by impregnation on the slide of paraffin sections of formalin-fixed tissue, again in silver nitrate, followed by reduction in hydroquinone (Warthin-Starry method). Alternatively, fluid may be expressed from affected tissues and smears made, these being examined by standard bacteriological methods, including dark ground microscopy.

Spleen

A large soft purple vascular mass of lymphatic tissue, situated between the stomach and diaphragm; it plays an important role in the metabolism and defence mechanisms of the body. Its functions are both haemopoietic and haemolytic. It is invested with a fibro-elastic capsule, from which extend numerous trabeculae which penetrate the splenic pulp and offer a supporting framework. The pulp consists of a dark red haematogenous mass, interspersed by small white rounded aggregations of lymphoid tissue, the Malpighian bodies or corpuscles.

Sputum

For the examination of sputum for malignant cells fresh specimens are essential; a suitable portion, solid or blood-flecked, should be selected and transferred by wire loop to a glass slide. It may be stained either by mixing the selected sputum with a drop or two of methylene blue and applying a coverslip; or by spreading an even film and, after alcohol fixation, staining by Papanicolaou, or by haematoxylin and eosin, or by a Romanovsky method. The usual safety precautions should be observed in the handling and disposal of such material in view of the possibility of concurrent infection.

Sterols

A biologically important group of substances characterized by the presence of four fused carbon rings, to one of which is attached a side chain which varies according to the particular sterol. They include cholesterol (q.v.) and its esters, the bile acids, the male and female sex hormones and vitamin D, and are widely distributed in the cells and tissues of the body, especially of the nervous system and the adrenals.

Sudan III

An orange-red disazo dye, widely used for the demonstration of lipids. Its behaviour and that of similar fat stains differ from that of orthodox dyes, in that staining is effected by the transference of stain from the solvent used (e.g., 70 per cent alcohol) to the lipid material in which it is much more soluble.

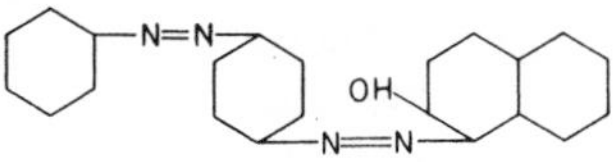

Sudan III

Solubility at $20°C$ is nil in water and 0.25 per cent in alcohol.

Sudan IV

A bright red disazo dye similar in behaviour and use to Sudan III, of which it is a dimethyl derivative.

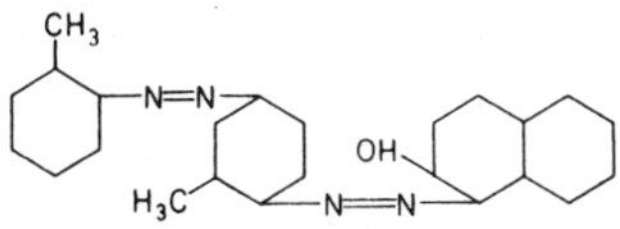

Sudan IV

It is sometimes referred to as Scharlach R or Scarlet red. Solubility at $20°C$ is nil in water and 0.6 per cent in alcohol.

Sudan black B

A lipid stain of the disazo group with rather wider applications than Sudans III and IV (q.v.); it is a useful myelin stain and can be used for the demonstration of Golgi apparatus.

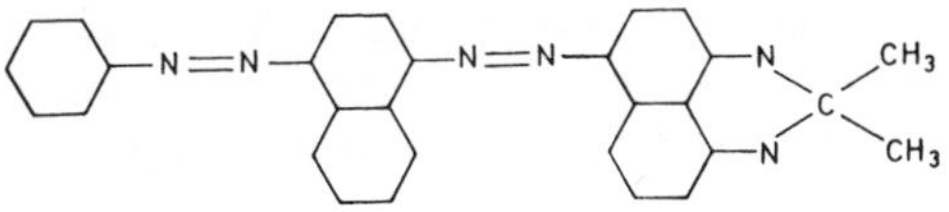

Sudan black B

Solubility at $20°C$ is nil in water and 1.125 per cent in alcohol.

Sulphuric acid(H_2SO_4)

A colourless, oily, highly corrosive liquid, odourless when pure but with a choking smell when adulterated with sulphur trioxide. Extreme caution is essential when handling it, especially when making dilutions; the acid should always be added very slowly to the diluent. Histologically it may be used as a differentiator, e.g. a 25 per cent solution in the Ziehl-Neelsen method for acid-fast bacilli, and as a test for (1) calcium, with the formation of gypsum crystals, and (2) cholesterol, sections being treated first with iron alum and then with a mixture of sulphuric acid and acetic acid or anhydride. It is also widely used in conjunction with potassium dichromate for cleaning glassware.

Sulphurous acid (H_2SO_3)

A solution of sulphur dioxide (about 6 per cent), clear, colourless, and with a suffocating smell. It figures in the Schiff techniques, being generated by the interaction of hydrochloric acid and potassium metabisulphite. The sulphur dioxide thus formed is utilized first in the manufacture of the Schiff reagent in its conversion to leuco-fuchsin, and in the technique itself as a reducing rinse for the removal of excess leucofuchsin which might otherwise be oxidized and recoloured with the production of false positives.

Supravital staining

That branch of vital staining concerned with the manifestation, after removal from the organism, of living cells by means of dilute solutions of certain dyes such as Janus green B and neutral red, whereby such elements as mitochondria are visualized. It is advisable that such preparations should be examined on the warm stage of the microscope. Supravital techniques may be of considerable diagnostic value in the field of haematology.

See also Intravital staining.

'Swiss roll' method

A means whereby a strip of tissue may be examined in detail, by the expedient of rolling it up in 'Swiss roll' fashion, tying loosely with cotton before processing, the cotton being removed at the embedding stage. The method is, of necessity, limited to those tissues which may readily cut into narrow strips, such as small intestine, aorta, gall bladder and dura, or even skin. By this means a strip of ileum 4 in long may well be accommodated in a 1 in square paraffin block.

T

Tartrazine

A bright yellow acid dye derived from pyrazole, and containing the azo chromophore. It is a popular counterstain especially in conjunction with phloxine as in Lendrum's technique.

Tartrazine

Solubility at 20°C is 10.8 per cent in water, 0.1 per cent in alcohol and 2.0 per cent in cellosolve.

Tattoo pigments

A series of coloured substances, of necessity nontoxic, and derived usually from mineral sources. They cover a wide range of colours and by virtue of their occurrence in the skin normally offer no diagnostic problems. Occasionally deposits may, however, be found in associated lymphatic glands, e.g. in the axilla.

Telophase

The terminal stage of mitotic division in which the paired chromosomes, having gravitated along the achromatic spindle towards the opposite poles of the cell, appear to coalesce, thus forming two concentrated chromatin masses each invested with a nuclear membrane, the individual chromosomes being no longer identifiable. The cytoplasmic membrane then becomes constricted and finally divides; the two daughter cells are separated from each other and form exact replicas of the parent cell.

Testes

Paired male generative organs, the counterpart of the female ovaries (q.v.). They perform the dual function of producing germ cells (spermatozoa) and sex hormones. These organs are ovoid bodies invested in a dense fibrous coat, the tunica albuginea, and are divided into follicles separated by delicate septa derived from the tunica. Functionally they are closely associated with the adjacent epididymis which acts as a reservoir for the spermatozoa, and with the prostate (q.v.) which furnishes part of the fluid vehicle in which the spermatozoa are transported.

See also Leydig cells.

Tetrazolium salts

A group of colourless compounds which on reduction yield highly coloured substances, such reactions being employed for the

histochemical demonstration of various enzymes. The colourless
parent substance, tetrazolium salt:

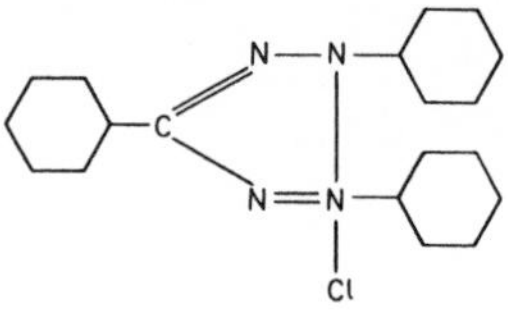

Tetrazolium salt

is converted by the addition of hydrogen into the bright red formazan:

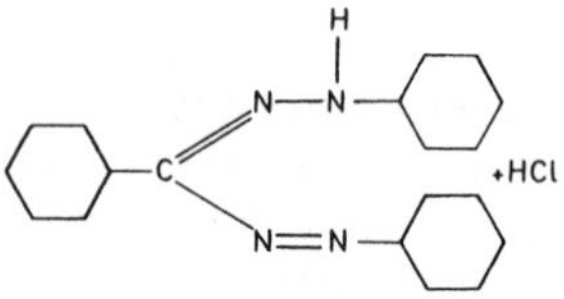

Formazan

    The reaction has found considerable application in the demonstra-
tion of dehydrogenases and diaphorases (co-enzymes I and II). Of
the large number of tetrazolium compounds, perhaps the most
widely used are neotetrazolium (NT) and nitro blue tetrazolium
(Nitro BT).

Thermomodule

    A device for producing low temperatures, dependent on a
phenomenon known as the 'Peltier effect', whereby a direct electric
current is passed across the junction of two dissimilar metals, heat
being emitted by the one and absorbed by the other, or *vice versa*
according to the direction of the current. The degree of refrigeration
is proportional to the amount of current, precise temperature control
thereby being made possible. Such devices are available in the form
of small platforms which may readily replace the chuck of the
standard freezing or other type of microtome. The technique has
obvious advantages over the older methods in that the use of carbon
dioxide cylinders is obviated, and also the accurate thermostatic
control enables large numbers of sections to be cut over a prolonged
period.

Thiazins

    A subdivision of the quinone-imine dyes characterized by the
chromophoric group:

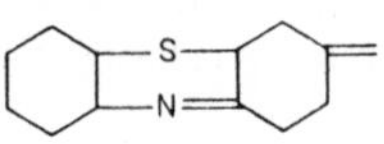

Thiazin

130

The important blue basic dyes, thionin, toluidine blue, methylene blue, and the azures are among its members. Methylene blue, apart from its use alone as a nuclear stain, is used in conjunction with eosin in the preparation of the Romanovsky group of neutral dyes which are widely employed as blood stains.

Thionin

An important violet basic dye of the thiazin subgroup of the quinone-imine series. Its generally accepted formula is:

Thionin

It has powerful metachromatic properties; hence it is of value as a stain for mucin, mast cells, etc., which are coloured red against a blue ground. It is also widely used to demonstrate Nissl bodies (q.v.), and in Schmorl's techniques for bone canaliculi.

Solubility at 20°C is 0.2 per cent in alcohol and 0.2 per cent in water.

Thymus

A soft pinkish bilobed gland lying immediately behind the sternum. It consists of small interlinked lobules separated by septa derived from a fibrous capsule. Each lobule contains numerous lymphocytes densely packed in the cortical areas nearest the septa and more sparse toward the central medullary core. The medulla also contains characteristic ovoid or spherical masses known as Hassall's corpuscles which are formed of concentric rings of dead or degenerate epithelial cells. The gland increases in size normally up to the age of puberty after which it begins to atrophy or 'involute' becoming almost completely replaced by fat in adult life.

Thyroid

A large vascular ductless (endocrine) gland composed of two lobes connected by an isthmus and situated athwart the trachea. Functionally its secretions control the basic metabolic rate and especially carbohydrate metabolism. The gland is composed of colloid-containing vesicles of various sizes which are lined by cubical epithelium.

Tigroid bodies

See Nissl bodies.

Toluene ($C_6H_5.CH_3$)

A hydrocarbon derived from tar oil. It is a clear, highly inflam-

131

mable liquid with a characteristic odour. It is employed as a clearing agent and is less toxic than benzene.

Toluidine blue

A dye similar in its chemical properties and applications to thionin (q.v.) with the formula:

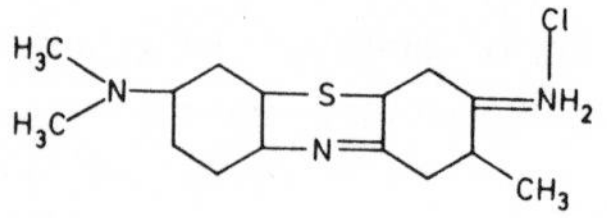

Toluidine blue

Apart from its uses which are dealt with under the heading of thionin, it is employed sometimes as a nuclear stain in rapid frozen or smear techniques where it is usually preferred to thionin.

Solubility at 20°C is 2.5 per cent in water and 0.5 per cent in alcohol.

Trichloroacetic acid (CCl_3COOH)

A colourless, very deliquescent, caustic crystalline solid, used as a fixing agent, invariably in combination because of its swelling effect on tissues; in Heidenhain's 'SUSA', for example, it accompanies formalin, mercuric chloride, sodium chloride and acetic acid. It is a general protein precipitant and has useful decalcifying properties. A 4 per cent solution of trichloroacetic acid is also used for the extraction of both types of nucleic acid (RNA and DNA).

Trichrome methods

A rather loosely-defined term usually taken to mean the Masson connective tissue stain and the innumerable variants that have been based upon it, by Masson himself, by Mallory, by Heidenhain, by Lendrum, and so on. Its meaning is often extended to include any three-colour (or indeed any multi-colour) technique such as Weigert and Van Gieson, Papanicolaou, etc.

Trypan blue

A vital acid dye of the disazo group, widely used to demonstrate cells of the reticulo-endothelial system and also the uriniferous tubules of the kidney.

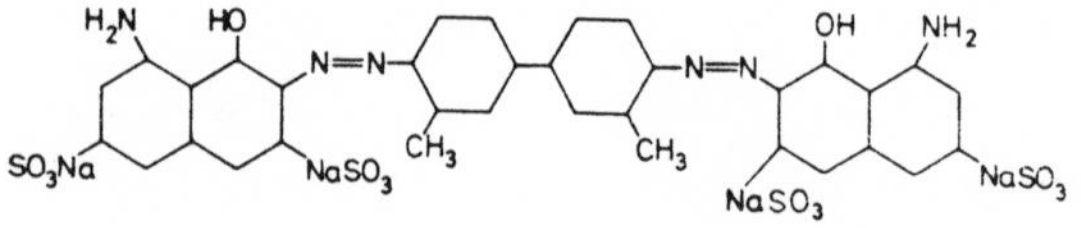

Trypan blue

Solubility at 20°C is 10.58 per cent in water.

Tweens

These are commercial detergents, which are water-soluble esters of long-chained saturated or unsaturated fatty acids with polyglycols or polymannitols; several have been employed in the demonstration of the aliesterases (q.v.). Those most commonly used are Tween 20 (lauric ester), Tween 40 (palmitic ester), Tween 60 (stearic ester), Tween 80 (oleic ester) and Tween 85 (ricinoleic ester). Of these, the first three are saturated, the latter two are unsaturated Tweens.

See Aliesterases; Lipase.

Tyrosinase (Dopa-oxidase)

One of the oxidative group of enzymes, it is responsible for the conversion of the amino-acid tyrosine into melanin and is widely distributed in animal and plant tissue. Its absence is regarded as a contributory factor in albinism. The demonstration of tyrosinase depends upon its ability to oxidize dihydroxyphenylalanine (DOPA) to melanin. This histochemical reaction is essentially similar to that which occurs *in vivo,* the only difference between tyrosine and DOPA being the presence of an added OH group in the benzene ring of the latter.

$$HO-\bigcirc-CH_2CH(NH_2)COOH$$

Tyrosine

$$HO-,HO-\bigcirc-CH_2CH(NH_2)COOH$$

DOPA

U

Ultra-microtome

An instrument devised for obtaining very thin tissue sections (5 to 50 nm) for study by electron microscopy (q.v.). Several types are available, all of them differing basically from the standard microtomes in the increased accuracy of the feed mechanism, controlled either by a modified micrometer feed or by a thermal advance system. Moreover, special embedding media are required in order to obtain such sections, resins and plastics normally being used. Glass or diamond knives are essential for this form of microtomy.

Unna-Pappenheim

A method devised originally (1910) in order to demonstrate

133

plasma cells, and employing a phenolized mixture of methyl green and pyronin in glycerin and water. It has found increased favour over recent years for the differential demonstration of ribonucleic acid (RNA) and desoxyribonucleic acid (DNA), the former staining red with pyronin, the latter green. In this connection its use has been further extended to the staining of Nissl substance. The behaviour of the solution tends to be capricious, owing to the unpredictability of the two dye components, and latterly attempts have been made to stabilize the stain by the use of buffer solutions.

See also Methyl green; Pyronin; RNA; DNA.

Uric acid (and Urates)

These compounds arise as the result of nucleoprotein breakdown by way of the organic bases known as purines. Most of the uric acid so formed is oxidized and excreted in the form of urea. Sometimes, however, aggregations occur, most commonly either as uric acid calculi or 'infarcts' in the kidneys, or as gouty 'tophi' in the joints. The substance so formed may be of variable composition and includes uric acid, monosodium urate and a double compound of both. The compounds are slightly soluble in water and highly so in aqueous lithium carbonate. They are insoluble in alcohol, ether and chloroform. Fixation in alcohol or Carnoy is therefore recommended; pretreatment in 6 per cent xanthydrol in acetic acid has been suggested by Oestreicher. Histologically their powerful reducing properties enable them to be demonstrated by Schmorl's reagent or ammoniacal silver. Confusion with calcium salts may be obviated by the use of control sections treated with 0.5 per cent hydrochloric acid in alcohol. Alternatively, a differential staining picture may be obtained with the Schultz method using carmine, methylene blue and picric acid.

Uterus

The uterus or womb is an inverted pear-shaped, hollow, muscular organ, lying centrally in the female pelvis between the bladder and rectum. The nulliparous adult uterus is approximately 7 cm long and, for the purpose of description, is divided into three main parts: (1) the fundus, which is the broad upper end of the body from which the Fallopian tubes arise on each side; (2) the body (corpus uteri), extending from the fundus to the neck; and (3) the neck (cervix uteri) which is surrounded below by the vagina into which it projects forming the vaginal portion. The body of the uterus is composed of smooth involuntary muscle (myometrium) and its slit-like cavity is lined by a special type of mucous membrane (endometrium) which is pitted with many simple tubular glands. The lower part of the endometrial cavity merges into the endocervical canal at a point

134

known as the internal os. The endocervical canal is lined by a single
layer of tall columnar mucus-secreting cells overlying cellular fibrous
tissue which contains numerous branched tubular glands lined with
similar epithelium. The external or vaginal surface of the cervix is
covered by non-keratinizing stratified squamous epithelium.

V

Vacuum embedding

A procedure, more correctly termed vacuum impregnation, often
incorporated in routine paraffin processing, whereby impregnation
with paraffin wax is expedited by subjecting the tissues to a negative
pressure of 400–500 mm of mercury. A thermostatically controlled
air-tight oven with an attached exhaust pump is normally employed
for the purpose, as the clearing agent and any residual air are
extracted more rapidly by this means. Cystic, fatty, and spongy
tissues, notably lung, are ideally suited to this treatment. It is
perhaps contraindicated in the processing of CNS material.

Van Gieson, Ira Thompson (1866–1913)

An American neuropathologist noted in histology for his picro-
fuchsin solution commonly employed as a stain for collagen and
muscle following Weigert's iron haematoxylin. It has, moreover,
considerable application as a counterstain in methods for elastic,
calcium, myelin, etc.

Verhoeff, Frederick Hermann (1874–   )

An American ophthalmologist who devised a useful technique for
the demonstration of elastic fibres in tissue sections. The essential
solution is an iodized iron haematoxylin, differentiation being
carried out in ferric chloride. The method is commonly employed in
conjunction with Van Gieson's stain for collagen and muscle fibres.

Victoria blue

Several different dyes of the phenyl methane group bear this
name with the designation B, R, or 4R. The most important application of this dye in histology is for the demonstration of astroglia,
and for this purpose the 4R variety is recommended.

Victoria blue

Vital staining

A term usually denoting any form of staining of living cells or tissues, and thus incorporating both supravital (*in vitro*) and intravital (*in vivo*) techniques. Some authorities, however, confine its usage to the latter category, and designate only the *in vivo* methods as vital staining. It would seem logical nevertheless to employ 'vital staining' as a generic term to embrace supravital and intravital techniques, which are themselves amply distinguished by their prefixes.

See also Intravital staining; Supravital staining.

Vulpian reaction

A name given to the treatment of fresh slices of adrenal tissue with dilute ferric chloride solution, whereby the medulla is coloured green, owing to the presence of adrenalin.

See also Chromaffin.

W

Waxes

In histology this term has a wide variety of connotations.

(1)   In lipid histochemistry it represents a subdivision of the simple lipids and refers to esters of higher (usually mono-hydroxy-) alcohols; they constitute, for the most part, secretory and protective substances such as beeswax, spermaceti, and lanoline, the only group of major importance in human histology being the esters of the steroid alcohol cholesterol ($C_{27}H_{45}OH$) (q.v.).

(2)   Paraffin wax is a mixture of hydrocarbons having the formula C_nH_{2n+2}, the number of carbon atoms ranging from 22 to 28. It is a white microcrystalline solid used extensively in the histology laboratory as an embedding medium. It may be obtained commercially either in slab form, in cubes, or kibbled (in particles about ¼ in diameter), with melting points ranging from $42°$ to $64°C$. A satisfactory paraffin wax should be of small crystal size and to this end additives such as beeswax and other fatty esters are often incorporated in its manufacture.

(3)   Water-soluble or carbowaxes (*see* Polyethylene glycols).

(4)   Ester waxes (q.v.).

'Wear and tear' pigment

See Lipofuscins; Brown atrophy.

Weigert, Karl (1843–1904)

A renowned German histologist with a remarkable diversity of interests. He has given his name to numerous methods and their associated staining solutions and reagents. Among the more note-worthy are his iron haematoxylin, his fuchselin stain for elastic fibres, and stains for micro-organisms, fibrin and myelin. His collaboration with Dr. Georg Grübler during the latter years of the nineteenth century is also worthy of mention, inasmuch as it resulted in the first serious attempt to produce standardized dyes of high purity for biological purposes.

X

Xanthene dyes

A family of dyes including the pyronins, rhodamines, the import-ant group of fluoresceins, and the phenolphthaleins. Among these, pyronin Y figures as a constituent of the Unna-Pappenheim stain for the demonstration of RNA, the rhodamines are sometimes used as fluorescent dyes, and the fluoresceins such as eosin and phloxine are extensively used as plasma stains. The phenolphthaleins are of little importance as histological dyes but include a very valuable series of acid—base indicators. The chromophoric structure which characterizes stains of the xanthene family is usually accepted as:

H (or benzene ring)

Xylene ($C_6H_4(CH_3)_2$)

A clear, colourless, inflammable liquid derived from coal tar. Three isomers exist, ortho-, meta- and para-, according to the relative positions of the methyl radicals. Commercial xylene is normally a mixture of the three isomers, metaxylene predominating. It is almost universally used in staining methods for the removal of paraffin wax and as a clearing agent in the terminal stages. In this connection, especially in celloidin techniques, a mixture of xylene, creosote, and phenol may be used. With equal parts of aniline it is used as a differentiator for fibrin in some Gram variants. It is occasionally used as a tissue clearing agent (antemedium) and has the virtue of rapidity; but it has a considerably harsher action than chloroform, toluene, and other agents. It is also the generally accepted solvent for the resinous and plastic mounting media. Its fat-solvent properties render it useful for cleaning purposes.

Z

Zenker, Konrad (died 1894)

A German pathologist whose eponymous fixative is widely used in this country and even more so in America. Its essential ingredients are mercuric chloride and potassium dichromate, to which is added glacial acetic acid immediately before use. This mixture constitutes an excellent micro-anatomical fixative and permits good nuclear and cytoplasmic staining. Numerous variants have been devised from the chrome-sublimate stock solution, by such workers as Helly, Orth, Maximow, etc., with a resultant modification of effects on the tissues; e.g. the replacement of acetic acid by formalin, as in Helly's fluid (q.v.), is recommended for fixation of haemopoietic tissues and of mitochondria.

Ziehl-Neelsen

The standard technique for the demonstration of *Mycobacterium tuberculosis,* it takes its name from two German physicians, Franz Ziehl (1859–1926) and Friedrich Karl Adolf Neelsen (1854–1894). The method, applicable to both smears and sections, involves staining the organisms with a strong heated phenolic solution of basic fuchsin, followed by differentiation, and nuclear counterstaining in methylene blue. Numerous modifications exist, none of which has in the least superseded the parent method. *Mycobacterium leprae* may be demonstrated by a slightly modified version of the method.